HAPPY, HEALTHY & SEXY

Lisa Sussman

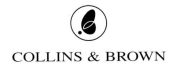

COLLINS & BROWN

First published in Great Britain in 2005 by Collins & Brown Ltd

An imprint of **Chrysalis** Books Group plc

The Chrysalis Building, Bramley Road, London W10 6SP

Published in association with
The National Magazine Company Limited.
Cosmopolitan is a registered trademark of The National Magazine Company Limited

9 8 7 6 5 4 3 2 1

British Library Cataloguing-in-Publication Data:
A catalogue record for this book is available from the British Library.

ISBN 1 84340 271 8

Project Editor: Victoria Alers-Hankey
Design: Penny Stock
Photographs: Michael Wicks

Colour reproduction by Anorax Imaging Ltd
Printed and bound by SNP Leefung, China

The information, advice and medical data in this book are only intended as a guide
and are not intended to replace appropriate advice from a qualified doctor. You
should consult your doctor if you are concerned about any health issues outlined in
this book. The author and publisher disclaim any liability from and in connection with
use of the information contained within this book.

HAPPY, HEALTHY & SEXY

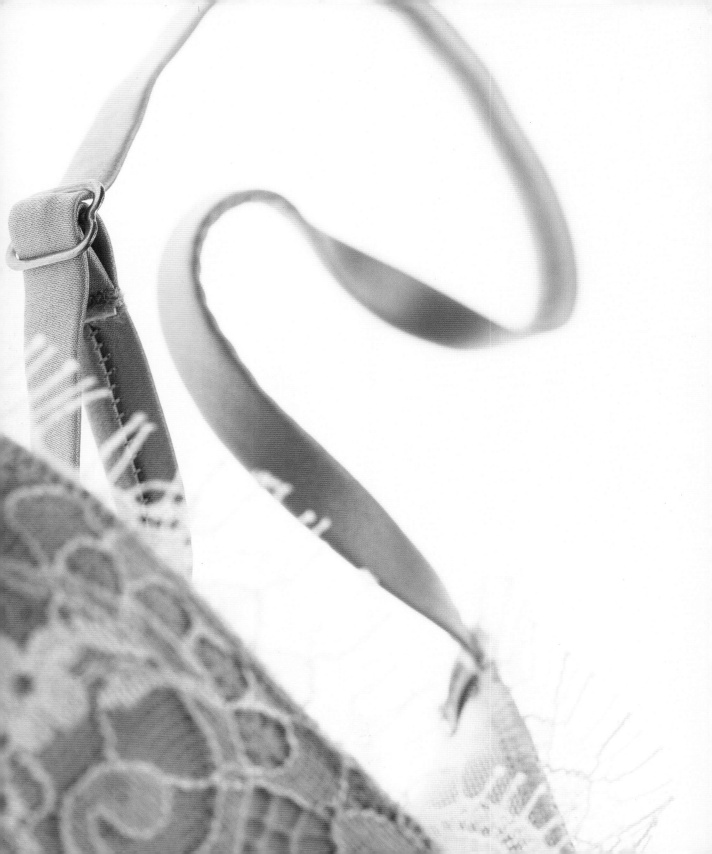

CONTENTS

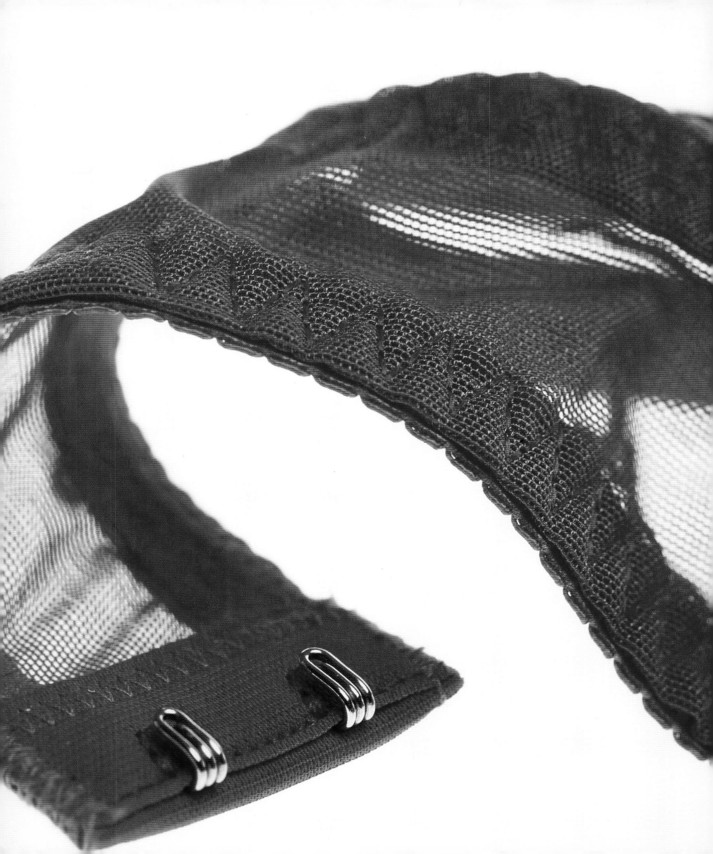

INTRODUCTION

So you don't know if this book is for you. Then answer this – what's the most important sexual health move you should make right now?

1 Read the instructions on your birth control.
2 Be able to name your parts from the areola to the womb.
3 Have a glass of red wine.

Doing all three will contribute to a healthier, sexier you. Here's why:

1 Most STI's are preventable. Pregnancy is virtually avoidable, if you use your contraception correctly. However, most of us just tear open the packet, pop the pill, stick in the shield and so on without ever looking at the fine print. But it is the fine print, my friend, which will keep you infection- and diaper-free.

2 Do you have any idea exactly where your ovaries are? If you're like most women, the answer is probably, 'Somewhere between my belly button and my vagina.' Why does being able to precisely ID your anatomy matter? Because it means that you know what how it looks and/or feels when you are in the pink. So when something is wrong, you'll know – and be able to help your doctor make a smarter faster diagnosis.

3 As for the red wine, countless studies have touted its health benefits. Apparently, resveratrol, a natural agent found in the grapes that make red wine has certain properties that help lower the rate of heart disease, prevent colds and check cancer. Now recent findings speculate that resveratrol may also have a preventative effect in the spread of herpes. And if your libido is running on low, other research has determined that downing any alcoholic drink can help increase testosterone (more so in women on the Pill) which increases libido (however, more than three drinks creates a reverse effect). Surprised? Of course you are. Amused? Hopefully. Curious? Then read on.

These days, most people know the basics of 'safe and smart' sex. However, what they know doesn't always carry over into the bedroom. For instance, this may seem shocking but a recent survey found that 40 per cent of women don't know how to use a condom correctly and 60 per cent say they would still have sex even if their partner refused to wear a condom.

Unfortunately, we tend to think of sexual health as something so mind-numbingly dull that's necessary to think about only if smelly slimy substances have begun dripping from your vagina or you have discovered a strange bump on your bottom. Wrong, wrong, wrong. Sexuality influences who we are and how we feel about our lives. Many of our toughest decisions in life will involve our sexuality. Since sexuality affects our lives so greatly, it is very important to be sexually healthy. This involves how you relate to your partner sexually and how you feel about sexuality in general.

Just look at the phrase 'sexual health' – the first three letters spell 'sex'. A linguistic accident? I think not. Staying sexually healthy is what keeps you sexy, happy and orgasmic. Studies have found that the healthier you are, the more you enjoy sex and the more you enjoy sex, the healthier you are. Which sort of makes staying in top-top shape sexually a no-brainer.

In this book you will find no-nonsense answers to questions you didn't even know you needed to know about your sexual health as well as all those things you are too embarrassed to ask your doctor and hundreds of health-related mysteries are explained:

- Detailed mouth-watering techniques for better, longer sex.
- How to stop condom abuse.
- What an orgasm feels like for a woman versus a man.
- When it's time to switch birth control.
- Whether you are fated to never have an orgasm or feel sexual again.
- Why sex sometimes hurts.
- What's the safest way to have anal sex.
- Why your vagina sometimes farts during sex.

Also included are the practical: how your body works, how not to screw up your birth control, how not to get pregnant, how to get pregnant, how to handle common symptoms (such as redness, itching, dryness, and discharge). And just for fun, I threw in the most recent information on contraception and new drugs and resources for sexual dysfunction and sexually transmitted infections, tips for safe and pleasurable sex, and everything in between.

To make things even more user-friendly there is a resources section at the end of each chapter that gives information on books, organisations and websites that you can turn to for more information on subjects that particularly interest you.

And just to keep you on your toes, throughout the questions and answers I've thrown in lots of quick tips and facts on everything from how many new curable STDs are contracted every day of the year globally (one million) to the medical term for getting off on armpits (Axillism) – and yes, you will be tested! There are quick quizzes and puzzles – treat these these as road-maps for figuring out how you can incorporate your new-found knowledge to make your own sexual life healthier and happier.

My mission was to draw upon the latest medical research while still making your sexual health something sexy, fun and interesting. Step two was to put it all

together into package that was easy-to-understand and informative to help you enjoy more sizzling and satisfying sex lives (translation: lots of blistering orgasms). In other words, this is the sexual health guide your mum never wanted you to read! Everything between these pages is doctor-approved (without the Latin). I spoke with leading health experts, read countless medical journals and deciphered stacks of studies to get the smartest sexual health advice out there.

If you're a hypochondriac or a natural-born swot, you might be tempted to read this book from cover to cover. But it can also be used as a reference book to dip into as needed – before you go to your doctor or even on a date, when you are worried about a specific health issue, as reference for a trivia quiz, during a sex-chat with your friends, or to make a point to your partner. So turn the page… and guarantee that the best sex of your life – and the healthiest – will always be your next sex.

LISA SUSSMAN

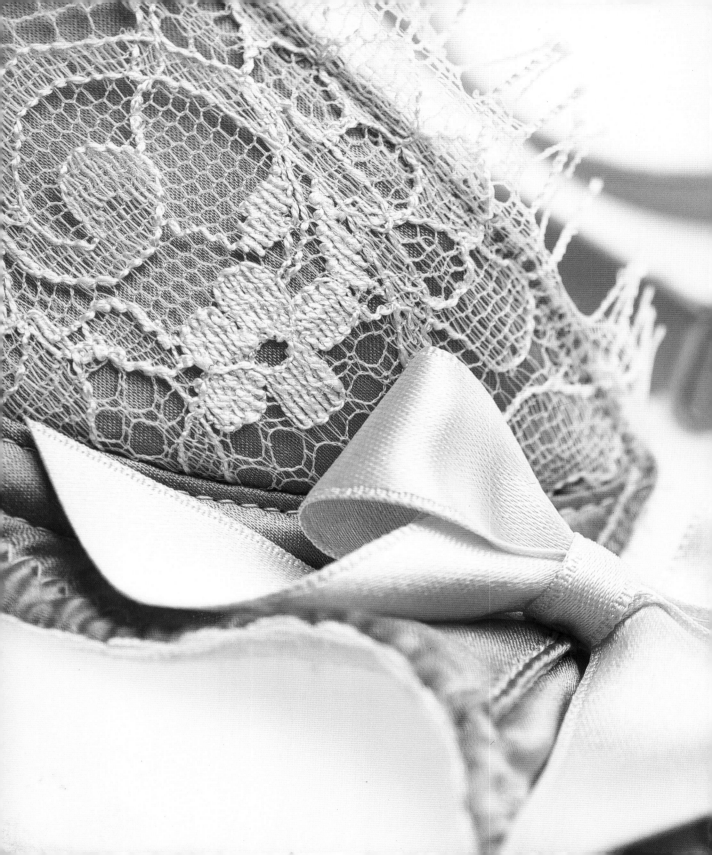

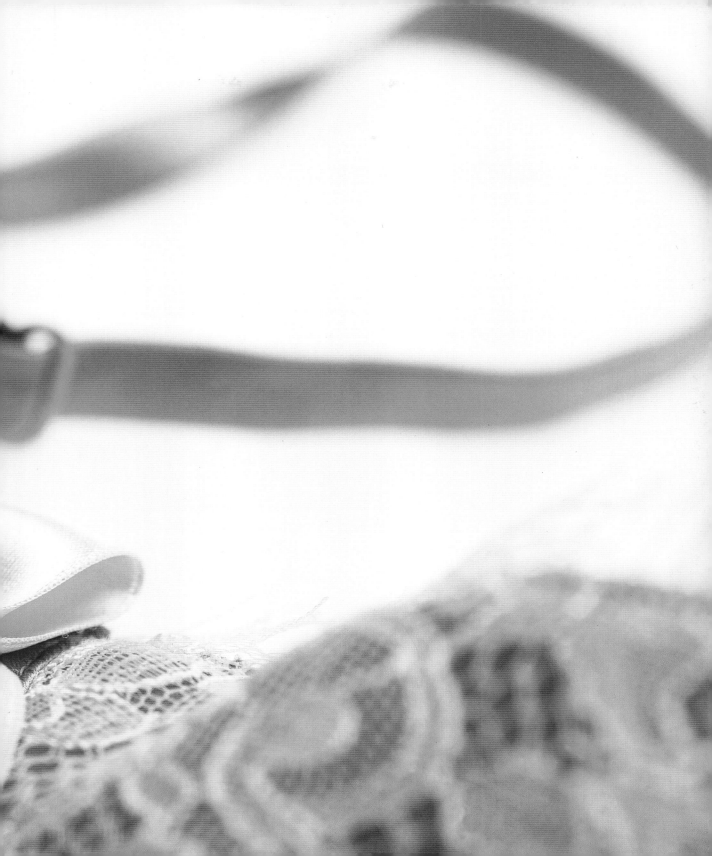

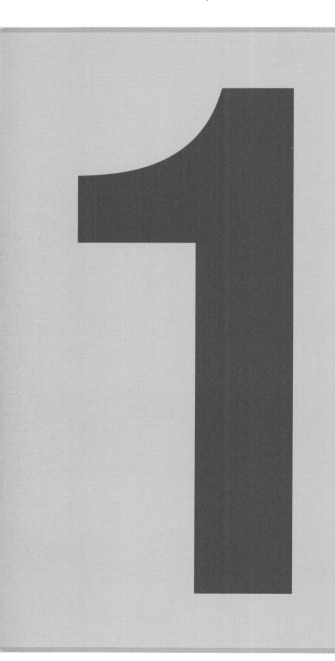

5 Healthy Breast Habits

(1) Keep abreast. Do a self-exam once a month.

(2) Cover up. Sun damage causes collagen to break down, increasing sagging. The V of the neckline is also a prime spot for skin cancer and age spots. So protect your cleavage with SPF15 or higher.

(3) Moisturise. The skin on your nipples is thinner and more vulnerable than just about anywhere else on your body (only your eyelids are more delicate). If yours are dry or irritated, soothe them with a cream containing lanolin (available from chemists).

(4) Do heavy lifting. Weight machines or free weights can help build up the underlying pectoral muscles, creating a strong foundation for your breasts.

(5) Keep your weight steady. Not just because weight gain is linked to breast cancer, but also because cycles of weight gain and loss can stretch breast skin, causing it to sag.

YOUR COMPLETE BREAST GUIDE

Everything you do and don't want to know about your breasts

No woman gets to her twenties, let alone her thirties, without having learned a few things about her breasts. But there are still a lot of surprising misconceptions circulating that can keep us from making the best choices about the way to take care of our breasts and knowing the difference between a painful twinge and something really being wrong.

BEAUTIFUL BOOBS

Breasts are as unique as snowflakes. No two are alike – not even your own set. But one thing is certain – breasts are more than just another curve in your anatomy; they are vital to your physical and sexual wellbeing. Which means that understanding about the care and feeding of your breasts is a key element in the satisfaction they give back to you.

What are breasts for anyway?

Apart from being kissed, fondled and generally adored, the basic job description of boobs varies, depending on what is currently happening in your life: your breasts can be sexual pleasure-givers, figure shapers, body accessories, health worries, self-esteem boosters or killers, pain causers, and baby nurturers. According to scientists, however, your breasts exist for two main reasons:

- They're feeders: Breasts are designed to nourish a newborn. In fact, anthropologists speculate that the cute roundness and up-tilt of a woman's breast evolved to prevent babies from smothering during breastfeeding. But rather than just being a milk delivery system, the breast is an active gland that, via an important neural hormone known as gonadotrophin-releasing hormone, might actually affect various systems in the newborn – including the brain (and thus, future behaviour).

> Breasts are essentially large sweat glands that have become modified to produce milk instead of sweat.

- They're sex organs: Breasts are secondary sex characteristics – it's their job to be alluring and appealing because this results in, hopefully, successful mating. They're sort of an upfront advert of the pleasures that lie within. Breasts have a special erotic wiring as well. During arousal, a rush of blood causes the breasts to swell and the nipples and areolas to get darker – much like what happens to a penis. The areola varies in colour depending on your complexion: it's lighter in blonde and fair-skinned people and darker in brunette or dark-skinned women. It darkens during pregnancy. Breasts, especially nipples, are integral to orgasm in many woman and – hallelujah – you've got two of them!

Why is one of my breasts bigger than the other?

Breasts don't come in matching pairs unless they come from the surgeon's operating room. In fact, nothing on your body matches. Your hands, your feet, even your ears are two different sizes. Generally the side of your body that you use more often (right if you're right-handed, for example) is slightly larger because more muscle develops on that side. In most cases, your asymmetry isn't noticeable to other people, even if it seems fairly obvious to you.

A difference in breasts is a cause for concern only of it's a new problem, that is, if your breasts were once pretty much the same size and one of them has suddenly inflated. If this happens, see your doctor to get your breasts examined for lumps and a possible mammogram to make sure that there isn't a growth – either benign or cancerous – in the breast.

Is it dangerous to get hit on the breasts?

In general, no – but best avoided. Watch the injury carefully, as a forceful blow to the breast can result in a breakdown of fat – which is not as good as it sounds. In fact, it can cause a permanent indentation. If there is extreme swelling or soreness, you will need to get checked out and possibly get an ultrasound to determine the extent of internal injury.

Why do I get breast zits?

Breast acne is not all that unusual – the skin of the chest is second only to the face in the number of oil glands. A dab of two of your preferred spot-busting remedy solution should help clear the occasional spot.

I have weird 'goose bumps' on my areolae. They don't feel like pimples, so what are they?

Those 'goose bumps' around the areola are called Montgomery's glands, special oil glands that are larger than normal and cluster round the nipples. Men have them too. Their job is to keep the nipple greased up with a substance called sebum. The skin around this area is ultra-delicate and can sometimes get dry or irritated. They are most likely to really pop out during sexual stimulation.

Ugh! There's hair growing on my breasts.

Don't worry, this is not a sign that your true career is in a fairground show. All women have hair around the areola, from one strand to a full head. The growth may vary through a woman's lifetime due to hormonal shifts.

You can pull them out with tweezers, but this can lead to ingrown hairs and infections. It is probably better simply to cut them off close to the skin (the hairs will grow again, so you will have to give yourself a trim regularly).

If you also have excess hairiness on other parts of the body and your periods are irregular, you may have polycystic ovary syndrome (PCOS) and you should see your doctor (see Chapter Three).

My nipples itch. What's going on?

It's most likely one of the following things:
- If the itching is worse at night and you notice grey lines around your breasts, you probably have scabies, a fairly common infectious disease of the skin caused by microscopic mites (see Chapter Eight).
- If your nipples are also scaly and cracked, you probably have eczema. A steroid cream from your doctor should deal with it.
- If you're a runner, you may have 'Jogger's nipple'. This is caused by friction from clothing, especially during long-distance running. Protect your nipples with petroleum jelly or surgical tape (available from the chemist) before exercising. A silk running vest

The Breast Ingredients

For all of the attention that they attract, breasts are really pretty straightforward — they're made up of three basic components:

① FAT

The amount and distribution of fat determines the overall size and shape of breasts. When women are younger, their breasts have less fat and are mostly comprised of glands.

② GLANDS OR LOBULES

These make milk and are arrayed in a circle around the nipple like slices of pie. But the slices aren't even (most glands are concentrated in the upper, outer quarter of each breast, near the armpit). The glands connect to ducts, which are basically a plumbing system of tiny pipelines through which milk travels to the nipple. During pregnancy and before menstruation, the glands in the breast expand and become more sensitive. After lactation and menopause, and as a woman continues to age, these glands shrink and the breast becomes mostly fat tissue in composition.

③ CONNECTIVE TISSUE

Fibrous connective tissue, which resembles the ropes of a hammock, surrounds and supports the glands. This, along with skin, is what supports your breasts. As breasts expand and then shrink during pregnancy and with age, the supporting skin and ligaments can become stretched out, resulting in breast droop — as you've probably noticed.

6 Things That Don't Cause Breast Cancer

① MAMMOGRAMS

It is true that in mega-high doses (we're talking nuclear meltdown), radiation can lead to cancerous changes in breast tissue. But mammograms expose you to only about 18 millirems of radiation per exam – the equivalent of two days of normal exposure to natural radiation in our atmosphere, or about four times what you'd get on a flight from London to New York. In short, the benefits of having a mammogram far outweigh the very minimal risks.

② CAFFEINE

There's no need to skip your daily java fix. Several major studies have found absolutely no link between caffeine consumption and breast cancer (the jury is still out on caffeine's connection with breast cysts).

③ DAIRY

In fact, several studies have found that women who drank more than three glasses of milk every day had a lower incidence of breast cancer. What's key is to keep it low-fat.

④ LUMPY BREASTS

If you haven't reached menopause, even a single lump is 12 times more likely to be something other than cancer.

⑤ ANTIPERSPIRANT

The myth is that antiperspirants block pits from sweating, causing a build up of 'toxins' which result in abnormal cell growth of cancer. But breast cancer is not caused by a build-up of toxins in the body. In addition, the purpose of sweating is not to rid the body of 'toxins', but rather to help regulate body temperature. It is the liver and kidneys that are responsible for ridding the body of unwanted chemicals.

⑥ THE PILL

This rumour was based on old research, but new, recent, large-scale studies have found that women who are on the Pill are no more likely to get breast cancer than women who have never taken the Pill and may even be at less risk.

is less abrasive than synthetic fibres. However, if you have an itching or flaking rash on or around the nipple (not the areola), it may be a sign of Paget's disease, a rare type of breast cancer that usually occurs in middle-aged women and accounts for about one per cent of all breast cancers. Over time, you'll develop oozing or crusty discharge or bleeding sores, caused by a cancerous tumour growing in the milk ducts inside the breast. So if your itching doesn't go away or you also have discharge, you need to see a doctor to find out if you need a biopsy. As with most cancers, early detection and treatment are key to survival and recovery.

My nipples leak – yikes!

Nipple discharge – also known as galactorrhoea – is usually no big deal. The cause could be:

- Certain medications such as tranquilisers, high-blood pressure medications, anti-nausea pills, some antidepressants, and the Pill.
- Pregnancy, even in the early stages.
- If you have breast-fed recently – after weaning a baby, it's not unusual to be able to express some fluid for some years.
- Inflammation (mastitis) around the ducts. This is linked with smoking, and may improve if you kick the habit. A course of antibiotics may help.

- Herbs such as nettle, fennel, blessed thistle, anise and fenugreek seed.
- Using drugs such as marijuana and opiates.
- Clothing that irritates the breasts, such as scratchy wool shirts or bras that don't fit well.
- Doing over-frequent breast self-exams.
- Over-stimulation of the breast during sexual activity – be gentle with those babies!

It's time to worry when your nipples start dripping spontaneously (i.e. not because they're being squeezed), in one breast only or if the discharge is bloody (whitish, yellow-green or even almost black fluid is fine). In these cases you will need tests. The cause can be anything from a benign growth to an imbalance of prolactin hormone to cancer.

If all the tests are normal, you can stop worrying, but your suddenly erupting nipples may be embarrassing (as well as upping your dry cleaning bills). In which case, it's possible to have an operation to close or remove the ducts that the discharge is coming from. However, permanently closing the tap may prevent you from breast-feeding later down the line.

> During foreplay, the female breast may increase in size by as much as 25 per cent.

I love it when my boyfriend sucks on my breasts, but recently he said he tasted something bitter. Is this normal?

Yes. Once in a while, nature has a way of reminding us what our body parts are really there for. Nipples are nozzles of sorts, and unexpected breast discharges are fairly common (see above). Ask your boyfriend to avoid sucking on the nipple itself (it can cause it to become dry and cracked) and instead suck on the areola – the pigmented area around the nipple.

I hate getting undressed in front of people because my nipples are flat. How can I make them come out?

Most women's nipples stick out about five to ten millimetres in the course of a day and expand to about ten millimetres longer and two to three millimetres wider during sexual arousal (yes, someone really did measure this stuff). Some women have nipples that are flat, but stand up to attention during sexual arousal, when they're cold or when a baby is feeding on the nipple. But about ten per cent of women have inverted nipples – nipples that are tucked into the breast, instead of being flat or sticking out. Both nipples may be inverted or just one. This may be genetic or just (un)luck of the draw.

> A nipple that suddenly becomes inverted can be a sign of a cancer underneath it, so you should see your doctor straight away.

If you're determined to become an outie, you could try:

- The Hoffman Technique: Place your thumbs opposite each other at the base of one nipple. Press firmly and at the same time, pull the thumbs away from each other. Rotate the thumbs gently around the base of your nipple. Try it five times each day.
- Wearing breast shields: These little suction cups draw your nipple out gently as you wear them at night for up to three months. Don't wear them for too long at first, otherwise the breasts may become sore, and don't continue wearing them for more than six weeks.
- Going under the knife: This involves a small incision on each side of the nipple, and the cutting of some ducts and tissue. The drawback is that some women cannot breastfeed after this operation, and it is very expensive (not available on the NHS).

ARE YOU WEARING THE BOOBY PRIZE?

More than 65 per cent of women today do not know their correct bra size. Here's how to custom-fit yourself:

- Take a snug measurement around your body, directly under your bust. Your arms should be by your sides, so get someone else to do the measuring).
- Add five inches to this measurement and you will get your chest size. Example: if someone is 29 inches under their bust, then their bra size is 34. (If your bra size comes out to an odd number, then just round up to the next even number).
- To get your correct cup size, take a loose measurement of the fullest part of your bust, again with arms down. Subtract this measurement from the chest one. If the result is 1 inch, then you're an A cup, 2 a B, 3 a C, and so on.
- Check the fit: Some women simply tighten the straps to make up for a loose bra, but that just results in the band rising up in the back – the band should be lower in the back than in the front. A band that is too high can cause neck, shoulder or back pain, and can leave indentations on your shoulders. When you buy a new bra, the band should be quite tight and firm on the loosest hook, to allow for stretching with wear. The bra cup should hold your entire breast, with no bit being forced out and with any underwiring resting on your rib cage and not on breast tissue.

Lately my nipples seem to be permanently stiff.

There's nothing like a spontaneous nipple hard-on to make you perky. The skin of the nipple is rich in a supply of special nerves that are sensitive to certain stimuli. When stimulated, the nerves send an 'Incoming Sensation!' message to the smooth muscle in that area to contract, which produces a nipple erection.
The stimulus can be physical (a loose shirt that moves back and forth over the nipple), or it can be a drop in temperature. It can even be a mental, like thinking about that sexy stud who serves you latte at the coffee bar. These special nerves are part of the autonomic nervous system, which is key in alerting the body that it's time to groove.

Some people experience them more often than others, but the bottom line is that what you are experiencing is probably one of those random weird things your body does that does not require further attention. Wearing slightly warmer clothing or a firmer, more supportive bra might help put your nipples at ease.

My nipples don't get erect during sex – is this normal?

For most people, erect nipples mean you're excited. But that's just one of many responses to stimulation. Breasts may respond vascularly – with skin flushing or slight swelling during arousal. So if you feel excited, you are, no matter how your nipples may act.

My boyfriend really loves to play with my breasts. Recently I have had red marks on my breasts and they seem to be getting worse. Should he leave my breasts alone?

Not unless you want him to. Most new red marks are some sort of dermatitis, whether they are on the breast or somewhere else on the body. The dermatitis could be either infectious (meaning of fungal or bacterial origin) or inflammatory (meaning that your body is reacting to something to which you are allergic).

Staying Pert And Alert

What will and won't work to reshape your bust and keep your breasts from heading south:

BREAST LIFTER	WILL IT WORK?
'Non-surgical breast lifts' using electrical (galvanic) stimulation to tone and lift the breast	Breasts do not contain any muscle, so there is no exercise that will improve matters.
'Firming' gels and lotions	These simply tighten the skin and so give a temporary sensation of breast firmness. Some claim that they contain elastin or collagen, the body's structural proteins. In fact, elastin or collagen applied to the surface of the skin will not be absorbed through it.
Surgery	This typically adds implants to maintain structure or removes extra skin and tissue from the breast and tightens and lifts the remaining skin. However, it is only a stopgap measure in terms of pertness – 'lifted' breasts will once again respond to the call of gravity as the skin and ligaments are gradually stretched over time.
Chest exercises	Sorry, not much point for breasts. Because the muscles in the chest do not support the breasts, exercises that claim to 'firm up' your chest area can indeed make the pectoral muscles under the breasts stronger and firmer, but they do not lift the breasts themselves.
A well-fitting push-up bra	Instant results. Always does the trick!

6 Things That Lower Your Risk Of Breast Cancer

(1) STAYING OFF THE BOOZE

Women who have one alcoholic drink every day up their chances of getting breast cancer by about nine per cent from those of women who don't drink at all. And the risk increases by about nine per cent for every daily drink consumed. In other words, regularly downing two glasses of wine a night increases your risk for breast cancer by about 18 per cent; three a night raises your risk by 27 per cent. So is it safe to drink at all? Yes, as long as you don't do it daily.

(2) STAYING IN SHAPE

Piling on the pounds can up your blood oestrogen levels and insulin levels, both of which are thought to encourage cancerous cell development. Women who gained more than 40 pounds during a single pregnancy face a 40 per cent greater risk of developing breast cancer after menopause. (Women who retained the added pounds after pregnancy were at the greatest risk, regardless of their starting weight.)

(3) STICKING WITH 'GOOD' FAT

While women who eat a low-fat diet have not been found to have less breast cancer than women who lard out, research has determined that eating monounsaturated fat (such as olive oil) may lower risk.

(4) GETTING OFF THE COUCH

There's plenty of evidence that going out and breaking a sweat can help lower breast-cancer risk, most likely because exercise decreases the oestrogen in the blood and may even increase your body's production of cancer-fighting cells. Aim for at least three 45-minute sessions a week.

(5) EATING YOUR BROCCOLI

Cruciferous vegetables (cabbage, broccoli, Brussels sprouts, cauliflower, etc) contain chemicals called indoles, which seem to induce the body to burn off the form of oestrogen that promotes breast cancer. Try to include these veggies in your diet at least two to three times a week.

(6) TAKING THE PILL DAILY

Early-stage studies suggest it may protect against breast cancer by stabilising hormones within the breast tissue.

Firstly, consider what material your bras are made of – lace can irritate the delicate breast tissue and some synthetic materials and underwiring can cause an allergic reaction. If this is the case, ask your pharmacist to recommend an over-the-counter cortisone cream.

The second possibility is that you are noticing stretch marks, which appear on the skin when you gain and lose weight quickly. These also occur during puberty as your body begins to shoot out in all directions. Sorry, there's no prevention or treatment for stretch marks, so don't waste your cash on creams that make claims.

A red 'sweat rash' under the breasts is called intertrigo. It may be sore and itchy, and you may have it in your armpits as well. The rash has a definite edge, and there may be some whitish material on it. It is usually caused by candida fungus or Corynebacterium bacteria, which likes to live in warm, moist places. If you are overweight as well as having large breasts, the skin crease underneath them is ideal for candida. It also likes skin that has been slightly damaged, as this makes it easier for the fungus to take hold. What to do if you have a red rash:

- To lift up your breasts, choose a supportive bra in a non-wired style (although underwired styles give good support, they tend to trap sweat). Cotton is better than a synthetic fibre because it allows sweat to evaporate. Wash it in a non-biological (non-enzyme) detergent and don't use a perfumed fabric conditioner.
- Wash under the breasts regularly and carefully, using a non-perfumed soap. Don't put any disinfectants in the water. Rinse well to ensure no lather remains in the skin crease. Dry thoroughly but gently – pat dry with a soft towel or use a hairdryer. Don't use shampoo in the shower – it may contain perfume that trickles down and irritates the area under your breasts.
- Stop applying creams. If you have been applying creams from the chemist, stop using them, even if they say 'for candida' on the label. You could have become sensitised to one of the ingredients, and the cream could be making it worse. Instead, simply follow the instructions above for two weeks, then see your doctor if the rash is not better. You may have to lose weight to eliminate it completely.

> In the USA, breast enlargement is more common than rhinoplasty (nose job) – there are about two million women whose breasts are not entirely their own (compared to about 150,000 in the UK).

Will my breasts sag if I burn my bras?

Contrary to popular belief, going bra-less doesn't mean that your breasts are destined to go bust. Bras do not preserve the shape or perkiness of breasts. Sagging results from a number of factors unrelated to brassiere wearing, such as:

- Breast size – the bigger you are, the further you are likely to fall.
- Age – breast ligaments soften and breast tissue reduces with the passing years.
- Pregnancy – the more you have, the more likely you are to droop.
- The laws of gravity – so let 'em loose.

I want to be bigger – are implants dangerous?

In the 1970s and 1980s, silicone implants had thinner walls than they do today, and were suspected of leaking their contents into the body, causing all sorts of havoc on the body's various support systems. However, no studies ever determined if this was the case. And silicone gel implants are considered to feel more natural than the alternative implants mixed with salt water (saline).

If you are still determined to upgrade to a bigger model, here's how it works. Implants can either be put beneath the breast skin (subcutaneous) and above the chest muscle or, for women with very small breasts or little breast tissue, under the chest muscle. The outline of implants inserted behind the muscle is less obvious than after a subcutaneous implant, but the breasts tend to be harder and do not move so naturally.

> The average breast size is 36C. The average model's size is a B cup.

Most women feel sore and get some pain and swelling. Breast sensation may be different and some of this may be permanent. It can take weeks or even months for breasts to 'settle' and look more natural. That's in the short term.

In the long term, you might experience leaks and ruptures. Another potential problem is capsular contractions. This happens when the body automatically responds to the implant by forming tough, fibrous scar tissue around it, usually in the first year after surgery. This scar tissue shrinks and the amount of shrinkage varies from person to person. In about one in ten cases, there is so much shrinkage that the breast feels hard and misshapen, and may need to be replaced. Also, implants make it difficult to detect breast cancer.

Another place you are likely to hurt is your wallet – cosmetic breast enlargement surgery is likely to cost about £3,500 for silicone implants, more for saline implants. For even more deflating news, bear in mind that your implant will not last forever. The average silicone implant lasts about 16 years, so you might need to raid your bank account at some time in the future.

I hate my huge breasts. Is there surgery that will make them smaller?

Breast-reduction surgery is a more complicated operation than breast enlargement with implants, and takes up to three hours. Skill is needed to make both breasts look the same shape. Within reason, the surgeon can remove as much or as little as you want, so you should end up with breasts the size you want. But this is a case of be careful of what you wish for –

> ## 5 Questions That Can Be Answered In One Word
>
> ① **What the number-one move I can move to keep my breasts healthy?**
> Self-exams
>
> ② **Are small breasts healthier than big ones?**
> No
>
> ③ **What is the darker ring that encircles the nippes called?**
> Areola
>
> ④ **If I gain weight wil be breast size get bigger?**
> Probably
>
> ⑤ **If you have a family history of breast cancer, does that mean you will automatically get it?**
> No

the operation is more 'final', as it cannot be reversed.

The surgeon removes a wedge of breast tissue and reshapes the remaining skin and tissue. The nipple will have to be moved to a new position. Usually you will end up with scars right round the nipple, in the crease line under the breast and along a line joining the nipple to the crease line. These scars take about a year to fade. The scar around the nipple fades first.

Each year, about 3,800 breast reduction operations are carried out on the NHS but, as big breasts are very rarely considered a serious medical problem, women usually have to wait about two years for surgery and may not be eligible at all.

> Not sure what normal feels like? Think of it like sticking your hand into a bowl of oatmeal – it's normal for it to be a little thick and lumpy. Breast cancer tends to feel hard as a rock.

Breast surgery, either to increase or reduce your size, may impact on your future choice to breastfeed. Talk to your surgeon about this; different surgical techniques can increase your chances of keeping your options open.

SORE, SWOLLEN AND OUT OF SHAPE

What kind of breast pain is a bad sign?

You may experience shooting pains during pregnancy or after a tough workout with weights when you've really worked the chest muscles. Seventy per cent of woman experience breast pain at some time and the good news is it's probably not serious. If cancers did hurt, of course they might be diagnosed earlier.

If your breast pain follows no monthly pattern and occurs in just one breast, it is known as non-cyclical breast pain. Rather than a heavy, bloated, tender feeling, this pain tends to be sharp or burning. The cause is usually simple, such as bruising from an injury, a sports strain, an infection such as shingles or a

Taking Your Lumps

Here are the three most common causes of benign breast lumps and how to deal with them:

WHAT IT FEELS LIKE	WHEN IT SHOWS UP	WHAT IT IS	WHAT YOU CAN DO
Soft, tender lumps	Usually in the second half of your cycle, after ovulation.	FIBROCYSTIC BREAST SYNDROME – benign temporary cysts formed by swollen ducts and milk glands. This condition affects more than 60 per cent of women of childbearing age.	Nothing. Since the condition comes and goes, there's no real intervention. You could try cutting the caffeine to help with tenderness.
A smooth hard mass that moves when you press it. It doesn't fluctuate with your period. You might be able to feel it during your monthly self-exam.	Common in the teens and twenties, less likely after age 40. It may grow larger during pregnancy or while breastfeeding.	FIBROADENOMA, a benign tissue overgrowth that can occur singly or in multiples.	Not much. It isn't usually considered a problem in young women, although your doctor may recommend a mammogram accompanied by an ultrasound to confirm the diagnosis. If you have a family history of breast cancer, you may need a biopsy.
A smooth balloon-like blister. If you push it, you can feel the liquid squish around it (although, it may sometimes feel like a hard immobile lump because of the breast tissue on top of it).	Most often in your thirties and beyond. It seems worse around your period – especially in the areas near your underarms.	Benign breast cysts occur when breast cells retain fluid and develop small sacs.	It depends. Cysts themselves are almost always harmless, but the presence of multiple cysts can mask a truly problematic lump, so your doctor may want to have them removed.

HOW WELL DO YOU KNOW
YOUR BREASTS?

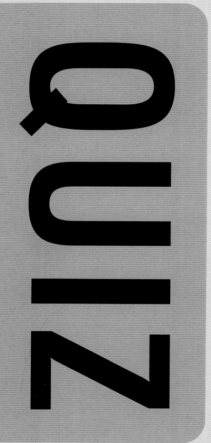

QUESTIONS

(1) What breast changes should be brought to the attention of a doctor?
a A lump or thickening in or near the breast or underarm area
b A change in the size or shape of the breast
c A puckering, dimpling or redness of the breast
d All of the above

(2) If your father's mum had cancer, you are at risk
True or false?

(3) Can men get breast cancer?
Yes or no?

(4) Which of the following has been shown to increase breast cancer risk?
a Underwired bras
b Antiperspirants
c Mobile phones
d Breast implants
e None of the above

ANSWERS

1 (d) All of the above. While it's unlikely to be cancer, any unexplained changes should be reported to your doctor to be on the safe side.
2 False. From what is currently known about breast cancer and genetics, the risk runs on the maternal side.
3 Yes.
4 (e) None of the above. The biggest factors for breast cancer are being a woman and long-term exposure to oestrogen.

breast abscess, a viral infection of the muscles between the ribs (Bornholm disease), inflammation of the joint between the front of a rib and the breastbone (Tietze's syndrome), a lung problem such as pleurisy, or even gallstones.

If your doctor can't find a specific cause, the pain is usually treated with non-steroidal anti-inflammatory drugs such as ibuprofen, or in the same way as cyclical breast pain.

My breasts get really sore and bumpy around my period. Is this normal and what can I do?

It's one of the side effects of being an ovulating woman. Before your period, your breasts tend to become lumpier and more tender with the surge in levels of the dynamic hormonal duo – progesterone and oestrogen. These hormones cause ducts and glands to enlarge as the body gets ready for pregnancy. The breasts may feel generally lumpy, but there isn't one particular lump. If you are unlucky, it may be so bad you cannot bear to be touched, are pain-free for only a few days each month, or have to wear a bra at night because it hurts to lie on your side.

● Wear a soft bra at night.
● Avoid jogging, aerobics or other high impact exercises.
● Make sure your bra fits correctly (see Are You Wearing The Booby Prize p.18).
● Try the Pill: it can stabilise hormone levels in some

5 Things That May Increase Your Risk...

(1) POSTPONING MOTHERHOOD
Women who have their first full-term pregnancy after 30 or never give birth at all are at slightly higher risk of developing breast cancer. In fact, the more children a woman has, the lower her risk of developing breast cancer – probably because she's not ovulating as much and thus her lifetime exposure to hormones is lower. Studies also suggest that breastfeeding offers protection against the disease, particularly against post-menopausal breast cancer.

(2) HAVING YOUR FIRST PERIOD BEFORE 13
Again, the longer you ovulate, the more contact your body has with oestrogen.

(3) HAVING A CLOSE RELATIVE – MOTHER, SISTER, DAUGHTER – WHO HAS BREAST OR OVARIAN CANCER
However, just because there is breast cancer in your family tree doesn't mean you will get it – only five to ten per cent of breast cancer cases are the result of inheriting a mutated gene.

(4) STARTING MENOPAUSE AFTER 55
Again, the later menopause starts, the higher your exposure is to oestrogen.

(5) EATING BBQ
Flame-grilling chicken, beef and fish can produce potentially harmful compounds in food called heterocyclic amines (HCAs) that may as much as double your risk of breast cancer. Marinate foods before barbecuing to protect meat from charring, so reducing HCAs, and keep BBQ feasts to a maximum of two per week.

(6) BREAST BRONZING
A tan is not a sign of good health and, although sunshine is a source of cancer-fighting vitamin D, it's better to up the D vit levels in your diet than up the risk of skin cancer by tanning. The V of the neckline is a prime spot for skin cancer and age spots. So protect your cleavage with SPF15 or higher.

4 Things Not To Try

(1) Diuretics don't work, because the pain is not caused by fluid retention.

(2) Vitamin B6 won't work and taking more than 10mg a day of vitamin B6 over a long period may cause nerve damage.

(3) Antibiotics are pointless; there is no infection.

(4) Progesterone hormone has been tried in tablet form and as a breast cream, but there is no evidence it does any good (apart from having a psychological effect).

women. (If you're already on the Pill, get your hormone dosage checked, as it may be too strong or too low for you.

- Cut the fats, as there is some evidence that high levels of saturated fats in the blood make the breasts more sensitive to hormone levels. Change your diet and avoid fatty meats, cheeses, full-fat milk, cream, butter and anything made of pastry.

- Load up on fish. Several studies have found that the fatty acids in fish such as salmon and tuna can regulate hormones, easing breast pain.

- Make a vitamin cocktail. For the few days leading up to your period, try a mix of 100 milligrams of vitamin B6 three times a day, 400 IU of vitamin E twice a day and up to 500 milligrams of Vitamin C daily.

- Massaging the breasts with ibuprofen gel has been reported to produce dramatic improvements. This is a non-steroidal anti-inflammatory gel, and is usually used for sprains and rheumatic pains. Researchers are not sure whether it is the drug itself that produces the benefit or whether it is simply the effect of the massage.

- Try avoiding coffee, cola drinks and salty foods for a few weeks to see if cutting the caffeine makes any difference.

- What your doctor can do:
Your GP may prescribe gamolenic acid, the active ingredient of evening primrose oil. Three to four capsules are usually taken twice a day for 8 to12 weeks. If it works, the dose is then reduced. It can sometimes cause nausea and indigestion, but has no other side effects. Of women who take this treatment, 30 to 40 per cent find their condition improves.

If gamolenic acid doesn't work and the pain is really severe (i.e. you can't function), the next step is hormone treatment to block the effects of hormones such as progesterone. This will work in about 70 per cent of women with breast pain. There are some side effects such as irregular periods, weight gain, headache, nausea, acne, oily skin and sometimes deepening of the voice. These effects can be minimised by taking the hormone drug for only the seven days before a period. It interferes with the effectiveness of the Pill, so you are advised to choose a different method of contraception.

Help – I found a lump!

Don't panic just yet. Breasts are naturally lumpy. Instead of being a big even pillow of tissue, breasts have several distinct components (see The Breast Ingredients p.15). Together, the glands, ducts, and connective tissue form a bumpy and uneven conglomeration.

When do I need to worry about my lump?

When:

- It's hard, fixed in place (it can't be wiggled around), irregular in shape and usually painless – it may feel as if it has fingers extending out of it.

- It doesn't change in six to eight weeks.

Both are warning signs that a lump could be cancerous and should be checked by your doctor immediately. You'll need a mammogram, sonogram or biopsy to confirm diagnosis – especially if you have a family history of breast cancer (see question below).

THE BIG C

I'm too young for breast cancer, aren't I?

You're never too young, though your odds are lower if you are under age 30. At age 25, for example, just one woman in 19,608 will develop the disease, according to the National Cancer Institute. By the age of 35, the odds increase to one in 622.

My mother never had breast cancer, so I'm not at risk.

Got breasts? Then you're at risk. In fact, 85 per cent of breast cancer cases are in women with no family history.

My family has a history of breast cancer. When do I need to get a mammogram?

It depends — if either your mum, sister or daughter (known as first-degree relatives) has had breast cancer, then your doctor will weigh up your other risk factors before deciding if you need to be checked under age 40. If, however, two or more first-degree relatives had had breast cancer, your doctor will probably advise you to get a mammogram soon and recommend a clinical breast exam every year if you are over 25.

For your own peace of mind, you will also want to learn how to do a self-exam.

HOW TO EXAMINE YOUR BREASTS

Lie down. Put a pillow under your right shoulder and place your right arm behind your head. Using the three middle fingers of left hand, check right breast for any lumps or thickening. (Reverse position to check your left breast.) Press firmly, examining your breasts in one of three ways:

- Use a circular motion; begin in the center and work out.
- Use an up-and-down line; start on the inside of the breast and work to the outer side.
- Use the 'wedge': divide your breast into a clock. Start at the nipple and work out to 12 o'clock, and so on until you're finished.

Check your breasts while standing in front of a mirror. Look for changes such as dimpling of the skin or redness or swelling of the nipples.

Also examine your breasts when you're in the shower. Soapy hands glide over wet skin, making it easier to detect changes.

You can also teach your partner to give your breasts a once over as he is probably as familiar with their shape as you are.

BOOKS

THE BREAST BOOK
by Miriam Stoppard
(Dorling Kindersley, 1996)
A comprehensive guide to breast health and care, containing advice and info on breast anatomy, self-examination, breastfeeding, the breast as a sexual organ, cosmetic surgery, developmental changes in the breast, diseases and their treatment.

101 ESSENTIAL TIPS: BREAST CARE
(Dorling Kindersley, 1997)
by Miriam Stoppard
This is an absolutely essential book for all women. It contains exercise tips and medical advice, disease and everyday problems accompanied by pictures and illustrations.

BREASTFEEDING: WHY BREASTFEEDING IS BEST FOR YOU AND YOUR BABY
(Celestial Arts, 2004)
by Susanne Arms, Chloe Fisher and Mary Renfrew
Fully illustrated, easy to read text and an upfront, evidence-based book that explains all you need to know about breastfeeding. A classic, produced by women who know the reality of breastfeeding.

DR. SUSAN LOVE'S BREAST BOOK
(HarperCollins Publishers, 2000)
by Susan M. Love, Marcia Williams
The bible of breast care books.

THE BREAST CANCER BOOK: A PERSONAL GUIDE TO HELP YOU THROUGH IT AND BEYOND
(Vermilion, 1996)
by Val Sampson and Debbie Fenlon
Written by a woman with breast cancer and her nurse, this book is a comprehensive account of options for women mainly in the UK. Sensible, practical and honest.

INFORMATION AND ADVICE

www.breastcancer.net
Features the latest news stories and medical journal articles on breast cancer research from a variety of online resources.

The Breast Care Campaign
www.breastcare.co.uk
Dedicated to raising awareness of benign breast disorders and is often the first point of referral for health professionals, enabling them to offer the appropriate support and treatment of benign breast problems.

Breast Cancer Care
www.breastcancercare.org.uk
A leading source of information on benign breast disorders. The group provides leaflets and information on benign breast disorders for both health professionals and the public.

BreastTalk
www.breasttalk.co.uk
Gives expert advice on how to measure your bra size and the best bra for your measurements for both the United States and the United Kingdom.

CancerBACUP
www.cancerbacup.org.uk
Europe's leading cancer information service, with over 4,500 pages of up-to-date cancer information, practical advice and support for cancer patients, their families and carers.

Mid-Atlantic Breast Cancer Information Exchange (MABCIE)
www.mabcie.com
A group of the medical writers and editors in the United States that goes 'behind the cancer headlines' to provide educational articles that explain the most recent advances in cancer research and cutting-edge trends in diagnosis and treatment.

The North East Valley Anti-Cancer Council of Victoria, Australia
Email: enquiries@accv.org.au
Website: www.accv.org.au
Provides information on breast pain as well as breast cancer.

Children's & Women's Health Centre of British Columbia
www.cw.bc.ca/
BreastCancer.org
A non-profit organisation that offers a broad range of medical, personal and practical information on breast cancer. It aims to help women and their families make sense of the complex information about breast cancer, and guide them to the best decisions for their lives. Especially helpful are the monthly chats, online discussion boards, and expert-reviewed original content.

The Coalition of Silicone Survivors (COSS)
www.siliconesurvivors.net/member.html
A non-profit organisation with over 5000 members worldwide dedicated to helping people become informed consumers. Get in touch for facts about silicone implants, articles, and a monthly newsletter.

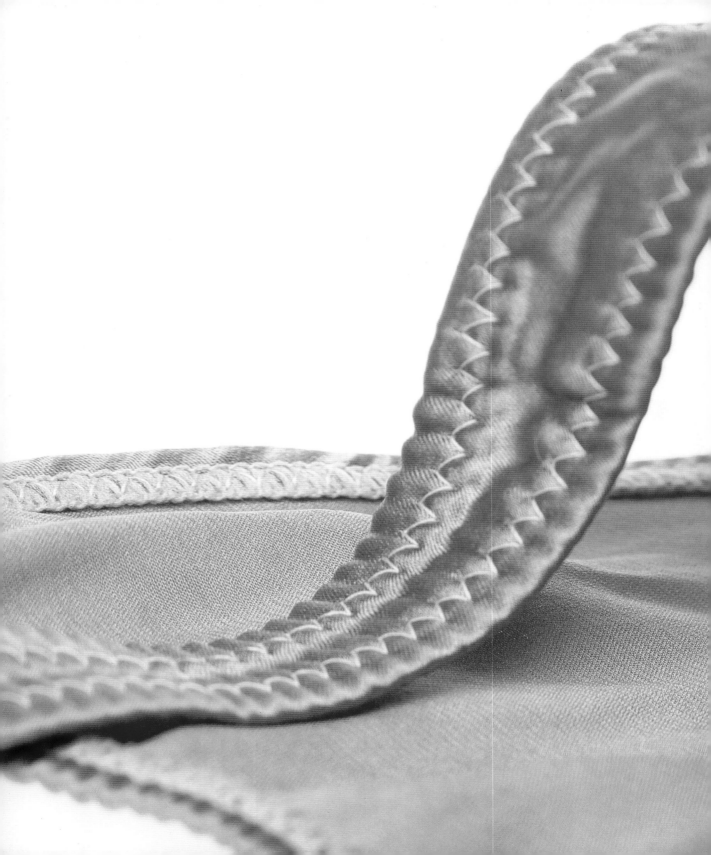

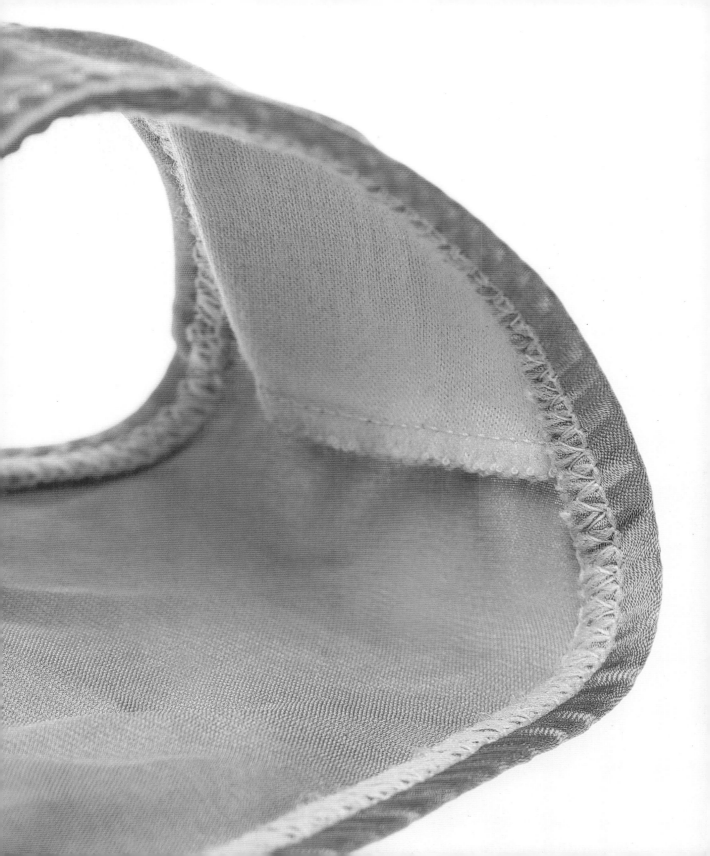

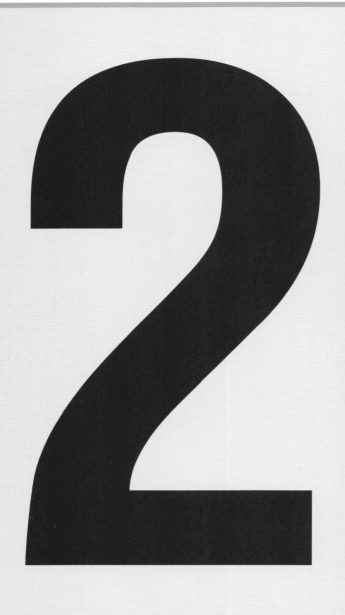

5 Healthy Vagina Habits

(1) Make a habit of peeing before and after sex. Urinating flushes out the bacteria that can cause urinary-tract infections.

(2) Stop using vaginal products. They can cause external redness or itching and derail sex. Let the vagina's natural clean-up squad keep things tidy.

(3) Have lots of sex. Regular sex (that includes masturbating) tones the muscles surrounding your vagina, intensifying orgasms, and keeps your vaginal walls flexible. Also, getting your vagina hot under the collar will trigger natural lubrication, which coats the vagina, protecting the walls from irritation.

(4) Moisturise. Women rarely think to apply moisturiser around the vulva, but there is a lot of dry skin in that area. Although you should never put moisturiser on your inner lips, it's safe to apply a gentle, hypoallergenic brand to the external areas, especially where your underwear may rub and chafe.

(5) Don't use spit as a lubricant. It's not as slippery as a water-based lubricant or your natural secretions and therefore can leave you vulnerable to small vaginal tears which allow infection to fester.

WHAT'S UP DOWN THERE?

Everything you do and don't want to know about your bits

The vagina is not simply a place for penises, babies and tampons. This four-inch (about) tunnel is also home to a variety of microscopic organisms that work together to make it as delicately balanced an ecosystem as a tropical rainforest. Left to itself, the vagina is one of the cleanest surfaces on the body. When everything is running properly, the friendly bacteria (called *lactobacilli*) constantly manufacture hydrogen peroxide, in effect churning out tiny bits of bleach to keep any not-so-friendly organisms in check.

However, as with other ecological disasters, we can usually blame ourselves when the vagina's natural balance is upset. We have unsafe sex, suffocate it in tight, unbreathable clothing, leave in tampons and/or diaphragms for too many hours, douche where cleaning isn't needed, take antibiotics which kill off healthy bacteria, mistakenly use non-prescription thrush cures when we don't really have thrush, and these are just a few of the ways we abuse our private parts. Read on for how to take the best care of your vagina.

HOW WELL DO YOU KNOW
WHAT'S DOWN BELOW?

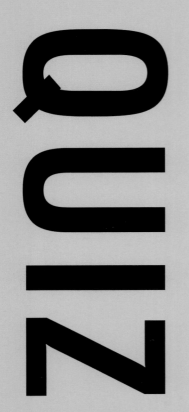

QUESTIONS

1 **Which of these isn't a part of the vulva?**
a The pubic mound or or 'mountains of Venus' – the rounded pad on which pubic hair starts grow during puberty.
b The labia or the vaginal lips.
c The clitoris, 'clit' or 'love button'.
d The vaginal opening and the area surrounding the vaginal opening (sometimes called the vestibule).
e The vaginal canal itself, which leads from the vaginal opening back to the cervix.

2 **The clitoris is just like a mini penis. True or false?**

3 **Which of the following is not a symptom of a thrush?**
a Vaginal itching, **b** Curdy discharge, **c** A fishy odour

4 **Can wearing a wet bathing suit for a more than a couple of hours lead to vaginal irritation?**

5 **The most common vaginal infection is:**
a Thrush, **b** Bacterial vaginosis
c Pelvic inflammatory disease.

6 **Should you clean your vulva with soap?**

ANSWERS

1 (e) The vulva consists of all of the external (or visible) female genitalia from pubic mound) to, but not including, the vaginal canal or the anus. The urethra, despite the fact that it is located mid-vulva (with the clitoris to the north and the vaginal opening to the south), is also not included as part of the vulva, since it is part of the excretory system, not the genitals.

2 False. There are some similarities: the clitoris is made up of blood vessels, spongy tissue and nerves, just like the erectile tissue in a penis. But they don't function in the same way. First of all, a penis has a many uses, while the sole purpose of the clitoris is pure sexual sensation. Secondly, the anatomy is different. The clitoris is more than what pops up under the hood. The part that you see is the glans, which becomes erect during arousal. Although this is the most sensitive part of the clitoris, it is just the tip of the iceberg. Just above the glans is the shaft (it feels like a hard rubbery cord right under the skin). It's connected to the bone by a suspensory ligament, where it divides into two parts like a wishbone, forming the crura. The crura extend about three inches on both sides of the vaginal opening (by the way you can't feel any of the stuff past the shaft with your finger). At the point where the shaft and the crura meet and along the sides of that whole clitoral area (aka the vestibule) are two bundles of erectile tissue called the bulbs of the vestibule. All of these parts make up the clitoris and they get all engorged and tingly during arousal. The crura and the bulbs of the vestibule are wrapped in muscle tissue and are partly responsible for the spasms that go on during orgasm.

3 (c) Thrush does not cause a fishy odour. The discharge will be odourless or smell slightly of yeast.

4 Yes. A damp bathing suit and a warm, moist, external vaginal environment make up an ideal setting for problems, effecting a change in the delicate pH balance of the vagina by entrapping excess moisture in this area.

5 (b) Bacterial vaginosis, caused by the overgrowth of organisms normally found in the vagina.

6 No. Skip the soap. And fling away the flannel. Perfumes and chemicals in soap can throw off the healthy balance of bacteria and yeast in your vagina and strip delicate tissues of natural oils.

BELOW THE BELT

What's the point of pubic hair?

There are a lot of theories, but no absolute answer. One thought is that it keeps our love triangle warm and cosy; another is that it prevents friction burns. A third theory is that it's a holding cell for pheromones, the come-hither seductive scents our bodies naturally produce to attract sex partners. Then there's the dust-buster hypothesis – it acts like eyelashes do for the eyes, preventing dirt from entering the vagina.

How big is the average vagina?

Most are about four inches. Remember that the whole area is designed to stretch to accommodate the head of baby. That's not to say that you should be trying to stuff the kitchen sink in there – a woman may be capable of giving birth but it's not something she wants to do every day. Still, most vaginas can make room for even a supersized penis. Here's how it works: as the vagina's owner gets aroused, blood flows to the genital area and sexual excitement causes the upper two-thirds of the vagina to expand and lengthen.

I have trouble getting a tampon up there, let alone a penis. Is there any way I can loosen my vagina?

Generally, that tight feeling is a logistics problem rather than a physical one. For instance, did you know that your vagina is tilted, so you can't stick the tampon straight up into your body? Or perhaps you're not waiting until you're sufficiently well-lubricated before attempting penetration. The problem can mean that you get stuck in a downward spiral – if you repeatedly try to have sex before your vagina is ready, the more difficult and uncomfortable it will be and the more you fear it will hurt, the tenser your vagina will become, which makes it hurt and so on.

My vagina is so loose, is there any way I can make it tighter?

Short of surgery (which runs at about £3,000 pounds a designer vagina), there is nothing you can do to make your vagina smaller. However, you can do exercises known as pelvic floor exercises to tone up your pelvic floor muscles (see Chapter Nine).

If your vagina feels flabby you may have a prolapse. The bladder, vagina, cervix and rectum are held in

NAMING OF THE PARTS

Picture two men talking about having sex…

Man 1: 'Sometimes I'm not sure what I'm doing, I'm all hazy about Down There.'

Man 2: 'No-one does. Just close your eyes and hope for the best. I think a girl just appreciates the effort.'

The miracle is anyone knows what's going on 'Down There'. Sex therapists say women understand so little about their own genitals that patients are routinely asked to examine them with a mirror. And what you don't know can't hurt you, right? WRONG. After all, you can miss out in every way – how can you know (and tell others) what pleases your body if you don't even comprehend what's happening? For example, you may think you're sexually cold when in reality, you simply have a hard-to-reach clit.

In fact, what most people don't realise is that women, with their mysterious private parts, have a far greater capacity for sexual response than most men could ever even dream of possessing. So get your compact mirrors ready for a quick lesson in your body's anatomy.

The vulva

We'll start with the vulva. Not a Swedish car, this is the external area of your love organs, covered with pubic hair. It protects the opening to the vagina and urethra. The latter is the small slit you wee through, below your clitoris and above your vaginal opening. Because these two openings are so close, sexual activity can sometimes lead to bacteria infecting the urinary opening.

Labia majora

The two folds of skin that meet in a peak form the labia majora (senior lips) or outer clitoral lips. These can be anything from pink to brown in colour. They are plump to help cushion both you and your partner during sex.

Labia minora

The *labia minora* (junior lips) or inner lips, are smaller, thinner and more sexually sensitive. They can be smooth or wrinkled and one lip is often larger than the other (go on – check for yourself). They join to form the clitoral hood, a loose lip of skin that completely covers your love button. Both senior and junior labia swell during arousal.

The clitoris

The clitoris (a Greek word, meaning 'little hill') is where it all happens. But most men, and many women, couldn't swear to its whereabouts (it's the fleshy knob at the peak of the inverted 'V' formed by the labia minora, in case you were wondering.)

With its wealth of ultra-sensitive nerve endings, your clit is a really touchy-feely organ. Even indirect stimulation through the labia majoris can lead to orgasmic joy.

The vagina

The vagina is a moist muscular tunnel that leads from the vulva to the cervix (more on that in a second). It's one-size-fits-all, with a two- to five-inch deep passage that can stretch to hold almost any penis.

There is still a lot of controversy (and even some relationship break-ups) over exactly where women experience the most sexual pleasure. The latest studies show 33 per cent for the clitoris, 66 per cent for the vagina and one per cent don't know. But what is agreed is the greatest vaginal high comes when the outer third (the opening and lower portion) is stimulated.

That's when your vaginal walls really start quivering with happiness and sweating little droplets of fluid. This lubrication is also what makes intercourse comfy and smooth.

The hymen

The hymen is a thin membrane that partially closes the vaginal entrance in women who have not had penetrative sex.

The cervix

The cervix is the opening to the womb. Ho hum, you say. But in the centre of this fleshy quarter-sized plug lies the os – an opening about the size of a drinking straw. It's through this 'door' that the sperm wriggle to set up shop in your womb.

G-spot

Yes, there is a G-spot (named after the lucky bloke – Graftenburg – who found it in the 20th century). This highly erotic pleasure spot is located on the front wall of the vagina about two inches in from the opening. There are even vibrators specially shaped just to reach this hot spot, but don't think there's something wrong with you if you can't locate it – it's tough to find and doesn't produce the same sensations in everyone.

The other organs of the reproductive system, the uterus and the ovaries, aren't considered part of the genitalia. However, they play a major role in reproduction.

The uterus

The uterus, shaped like an upside-down pear, is a muscular organ located in the pelvis between the bladder and the rectum. It has an internal cavity into which leads the cervical canal and the two openings in the upper portion leading to the fallopian tubes, right and left. The lining of the cavity is called the endometrium. This thickens during menstruation. The uterus then sheds the thickened lining (i.e. menstrual blood) along with the unfertilised egg.

The ovaries

The ovaries, located on either side of the pelvis, are a regular 24-hour breeding factory, producing the sex hormones oestrogen and progesterone as well as releasing egg cells once a month. A woman is born with about 500,000 egg cells and about 500 of these make it through puberty.

The anus

Finally, nearby and Down There, is also the anus, the opening to your rectum. Your bowel movements (faeces) exit the body through the anus. It is not dirty, because faeces are not stored there or in your rectum. Only trace amounts of faeces may remain there. Although not part of the baby-making equipment, it is considered an erogenous zone. Some women enjoy having their anus touched, rubbed or licked, or even anal intercourse (remember this can be highly risky if you or your partner has an STD, see Chapters Six and Eight).

position by the pelvic floor muscles that stretch across the pelvis. If these muscles are weak, the bladder and/or rectum can lean towards the vagina and press on it, or the womb may sag downwards. This is unusual in younger women. Treatment for prolapse is really surgery. The surgeon cuts away loose parts of the vagina and strengthens the supporting tissues. You might be given a ring pessary (a small device similar to a cervical cap or diaphragm) to support the vagina until surgery takes place. The doctor will fit the pessary and it will be checked every six months.

> Porn photos are often airbrushed so that the labia look smaller.

The inner lips of my vagina seem huge. Is this normal?

Like lipstick, vaginal lips come in all shapes, sizes and colours. They can be brown, pink, rose or plum-coloured. They can be fat or skinny, long or short, straight or slightly curved. No two pairs of lips look exactly alike. Sometimes the inner lips are bigger than the outer lips. Sometimes one lip is slightly larger than the other. This is perfectly normal: it's a genetic quirk, just like having a mole on your upper lip or curly hair. You can get cosmetic surgery to trim, enhance or simply give a facelift to your labial region but there is rarely a medical reason to do so and it costs a few thousand pounds per operation.

My clitoris recently began hurting so much that I can't bear to be touched. What's going on?

A brief anatomy lesson can help explain why you're switching from 'Aaah!' to 'Ouch!' The shaft of the clitoris is covered with a little hood, a fold of skin that is actually the upper part of the labia. The hood seems to protect the clitoris from too much direct stimulation; it contains glands that produce a lubricating juice called sebum, which allows it to slide smoothly back

and forth. And this might the source of your problem. When sebum accumulates, it turns into a white, cheese-like substance called smegma (no, it's not just a guy thing). Smegma, in turn, if not washed away with frequent bathing, can harden and rub between the hood and the shaft – think a grain of sand under an eyelid! An irritated clitoris can produce incredible pain at the merest movement, so tight jeans or pressure from sex can be excruciating. Accumulations of smegma can also cause the skin of the hood to stick to the shaft. These clitoral adhesions can cause pain and irritation as well.

Usually, frequent bathing and good hygiene can prevent or resolve this problem, but some women may have narrow openings to their clitoral hood that make it harder to wash away built-up secretions. If you have recurrent episodes of clitoral pain, you may want to try soaking in a steamy tub and gently move the skin around the clitoris back and away from the glans – but whatever you do, don't tug or forcibly retract the hood since this can cause further pain and irritation. These gentle stretches can, over time, widen the opening of the hood, allowing more freedom of movement for both pleasure and washing.

For a few women, 'do-it-yourself' measures are not enough. Gynaecologists might remove adhesions and/or stretch the opening of the clitoral hood after using a local anaesthetic to numb the genital region.

My clitoris seems huge: lovers have commented on its size.

No need to worry. Your clitoris may be bigger than the girl's next door. Sometimes adrenal glands produce hormones during foetal development that cause women to be born with a larger clitoris. However, this doesn't upset its function, as the purpose of the clitoris is to give pleasure. So just think of your XXL as a bigger pleasure-provider.

Is there any reason for a hymen?

The tissue helps keep germs and dirt out of the vagina at the embryo stage of development. But there is no such thing as an 'intact' hymen. Hymens vary in shape, size, and thickness. Some surround the entire vaginal entrance, with an open space in the centre (called an annular hymen); others appear open with a thin line of skin down the middle (a septate hymen).

Most hymens don't fully cover the vaginal entry, allowing menstrual fluid to leave the body. In rare instances, the hymen can be thick, covering the entire vaginal opening (an imperforate hymen). This kind of hymen may not allow a woman to menstruate, have penetration during sexual activity, or have anything inserted into her vagina. Often, a doctor can correct this with a simple incision (and should – as the vagina will fill with blood that can back up into the uterus).

A hymen can also be stretched or torn by fingers, tampons, masturbation, even during a gynaecological exam or vigorous physical movement such as horse-riding.

> The clitoris has 8,000 nerve endings, making it too sensitive to touch directly for some women.

I have some sort of blood blister on my inner labia. It doesn't hurt, but how should I get rid of it?

It sounds as if you broke a blood vessel in the vicinity, which can cause a blood blister. Have you gone on a strenuous bike trip lately? Or had some type of traumatic fall that landed you on your groin? Anything of this nature could have given you the blood blister.

The best thing to do is nothing. Like most other blisters, this one should go away in three to six weeks by itself. If your blister persists beyond six weeks or gets bigger after the first day, go to your doctor immediately. Your Bartholin's glands may be infected, especially if it gets painful. Bartholin's are almost invisible glands on each of the vaginal walls that produce the fluids that lubes the vulva's inner lips and eases penetration. Sometimes the opening of one of the glands can become blocked, causing a cyst. Your doctor may want to drain the cyst altogether by inserting a small tube (called a catheter) into the gland or by making an incision directly into the gland itself.

Is it possible to have genital acne?

No, but you won't necessarily be able to tell the difference between that and what you can get. You may have hidradenitis suppurativa – a mouthful that essentially means your sweat glands are blocked on and around the outside genitals. You can also develop folliculitis, an infection in the skin's pores, in the groin. Either condition can cause pimply lesions that mimic acne. Using an antibacterial cleanser may help clear the bumps, but check with a doctor if it doesn't clear up in about a month (or immediately if you have any reason to think you have been exposed to a sexually transmitted infection).

> Genital herpes and warts can also cause bumps and pimple-like sores around the bum (see Chapter Eight for more information).

What are fibroids?

These are common, benign tumours in the uterus that most women develop during the course of a lifetime (also called myomas, fibromyomas, or leiomyomas). For most, fibroids present no problems. But an unlucky 10 to 20 per cent of women suffer severe symptoms: heavy menstrual bleeding, pelvic pain and pressure, frequent urination, and abdominal distension. Sometimes they cause infertility by blocking the fallopian tubes or by distorting the shape of the uterus. Large fibroids can also cause pain in the lower back or abdomen. If you are pregnant, they can block the birth canal during delivery.

Some fibroids grow very slowly indeed. Others spread quickly, all at once. Only one fibroid may develop or they can grow in clusters or groups. Some are as small as a pea, while others expand to reach the size of a melon.

To halt fibroid growth, a doctor can prescribe a contraceptive that reduces the amount of oestrogen in the body. If this fails and the growth runs rampant, more drastic measures are called for, such as a hysterectomy (see What's Giving You A Pain? p.54).

A hysterectomy is the only treatment that permanently removes fibroids. However, you do have

CALL YOUR DOCTOR NOW CHECKLIST

If a cyst is larger than two inches across or you start experiencing any of the following symptoms, it may be interfering with your reproductive system and need to be removed. Call your doctor if you have:

- A sense of fullness in your abdomen.
- Swelling and/or a sudden sharp pain in your lower abdomen.
- Severe abdominal pain with a fever and sometimes vomiting.
- Pain during sex.
- Painful, irregular or delayed periods.

other less-freak-you-out options. Yes, the fibroids may return but it can take years. Look at the following:

- Myometomy: Less drastic surgery than a hysterectomy, this removes the fibroid but keeps the uterus fully functioning (i.e. capable of childbearing).
- Myolysis: A laparoscopic procedure in which an electric current is repeatedly applied to each tumour, destroying the fibroids.
- Lupron: Used in women who have excessive bleeding, this synthetic hormone shuts down the ovaries, depriving fibroids of the oestrogen that makes them grow. Unfortunately, it can cause artificial menopause so it can be taken for only three to six months.
- RU-486: Also known as mifepristone, it blocks progestins, the hormones required to increase the blood supply which is needed by fibroids to grow.
- Radiofrequency ablation: Treatment for fibroids using heat. As it's done through a laparoscope and requires just two small abdominal incisions, it's less invasive that the usual surgical approaches.

- Uterine artery embolisation (UAW): Shrinks a fibroid by cutting off its blood supply rather than removing it surgically. An incision is made in the groin and, using a thin tube called a catheter, polyvinyl alcohol (plastic) particles are permanently injected into the arteries to plug them and prevent blood from 'feeding' the fibroid.

I've just been diagnosed with a cyst. What does it mean?

Think pimples, except for the location of course. Unfortunately skin astringents are not going to help you here, though.

Cysts are quite common among women under 30 years of age, and about 95 per cent of them are benign. Several types exist, and they can range in size from pea to orange size:

- Vaginal inclusion cysts are the most common type of cyst found in the vagina. They pop up if the vaginal wall is damaged in some may – maybe after a gynaecological vaginal procedure, when the vaginal lining doesn't heal to its usual baby-skin smoothness.
- Gartner's duct cysts develop in the space occupied by the – surprise! – Gartner's duct, usually on the side walls of the vagina. It's one of those things we don't need after we're born. Portions of the duct may collect fluid and create cysts.
- Cervical cysts are caused by a blockage of the mucus-producing glands.
- Ovarian cysts are found on the ovaries, the small organs on either side of the uterus that produce female sex hormones and release an egg during the menstrual cycle. Most vanish after one or two cycles.

Since cysts rarely have symptoms, they are usually found during a routine pelvic examination. And because they're relatively harmless, you may as well live with them (see Call Your Doctor Now Checklist, opposite).

> A fibroid should be checked by a doctor regularly after it first appears, to make sure it's not growing rapidly.

Can ovarian cysts cause infertility?

Probably not. Ovarian cysts are a fairly common and harmless swelling of one or both ovaries. They can either be fluid-filled or solid benign tumours. About 95 per cent of them are benign. Many women develop cysts at specific times in their menstrual cycle. Most shrink and disappear on their own in a few weeks. You're most likely to get them during your reproductive years (between puberty and the menopause) when the ovaries are in high gear making ova (eggs). Clues include:

- Some change in your periods, including shorter or longer periods, missed periods, and/or spotting between periods.

> Birth control pills control the growth of some cysts, which improves symptoms and prevents the formation of new

- Pelvic pain or ache, especially during sexual intercourse or at the start or finish of your period.
- Feelings of nausea or queasiness.
- Breast tenderness.

However, small, low profile cysts may cause no symptoms at all, and may only be located during routine pelvic exams. If a cyst does not disappear within two menstrual cycles, or if it is larger than two inches, or if you're over 40 years old, your doctor may want you to have ultrasound scanning or laparoscopy (a method of examination using an endoscope, sort of an internal periscope) to look at the cyst more closely, determine its size and position, and a correct diagnosis. Benign cysts can sometimes be treated with hormone therapy, stress reduction techniques, acupuncture, dietary modifications and/or herbal remedies. Other cysts may have to be removed surgically if they are causing you undue discomfort or if they are interfering with normal ovarian and reproductive functioning.

DRIPS AND LEAKS

I seem to have a discharge all the time. Is this normal?

Probably, but possibly not. Being a woman can be a pretty messy business, and not just once a month either. The vagina is a self-cleansing organ. Its discharge of mucous secreted from the walls of the vagina and neck of the cervix has several purposes: cleaning and moistening the vagina and helping to prevent and fight infections. The body usually produces about a teaspoon per day, but this can increase mid-cycle (during ovulation), if you're on the Pill or use an intrauterine device (IUD), and during pregnancy. Being aroused will also get your vaginal juice factory pumping, because two glands near the vaginal opening (the Bartholin's glands) secrete additional mucus to act as a lubricant. Your discharge may be clear or milky white (it looks yellow when it dries).

You only need to worry if the discharge changes significantly – it smells, turns green or yellow or resembles cottage cheese, if you itch, or if there's vaginal redness and irritation. Any of these mean you could have an infection (see What's Dripping? p.42).

I get soaking wet during sex. Is this just normal sex fluid?

If your wetness is happening when you orgasm, you may be ejaculating. This is something women can do (see Chapter Four).

There are also people of both sexes who pee a little when highly aroused; and then there are people who are quite regularly wet when sexually aroused. Perhaps you use an IUD – any type of foreign body in the uterus can increase vaginal fluids. Or if you have oral sex, this might be causing your discharge as your vagina tries to flush out the germs invading from your lover's mouth and throat.

> A woman can be fertile with only one ovary, or with even one part of an ovary.

What's Dripping?

Here's how to decode your discharge.

DISCHARGE	IS THERE ITCHING?	COULD BE	TREATMENT
Thick and white	No	Your normal cycle	Riding it out
Thick and white, resembles cottage cheese	Yes	Candidiasis – aka thrush	Antifungal cream or suppositories
Smelly, frothy, yellowish-green, sore vulva and may be painful to pee and have sex.	Yes	Trichomoniasis	see Chapter Eight
Smelly, greenish-yellow	No	Gonorrhoea	see Chapter Eight
Smelly, greyish white	No	Forgotten tampon	Removing a forgotten tampon as soon as possible. Then, if your discharge continues for more than a couple of days, see your doctor.
Off-white, yellow or greyish watery or foamy discharge accompanied by a fishy smell.	None to mild	Bacterial vaginosis/BV (see The Big Stink on p.44)	Topical or oral antibiotics

In short, your discharge is likely to be normal. In which case, tell your lover you're just hot and juicy – and keep a towel near the bed to soak up any floods.

I leak pee when I am exercising and sometimes even during sex. What can I do?

You're in good company. According to a recent study, leaking affects one in ten women. Women who have gone through childbirth are most prone. It seems that the nerves can be stretched and bruised during the delivery, and they are unable to make the pelvic floor work after the birth. As a result, the muscles become lazy and weak.

Carrying extra weight also puts stress on the pelvic floor muscles. Certain drugs can relax the pelvic floor around the ring of muscles at the neck of the bladder, making leakage more likely. The most common culprits are some blood pressure medications (particularly alpha-blockers such as prazosin and doxazosin), fluoxetine (Prozac) and muscle-relaxant drugs. High amounts of caffeine and/or smoking have also been linked to the leakage. Some women are just born with a weak pelvic floor.

Pelvic floor exercises are the best remedy (see Chapter Nine). Severe cases may need surgery.

> Each vagina has its own unique smell, which can range from salty to musky.

I recently had a lot of sex with my boyfriend. Now I notice that I have a burning sensation when I pee. Could the two be related?

Say hello to honeymoonitis. This oh-so-painful problem is the most common of UTIs (urinary tract infections). UTIs strike when bacteria such as E.coli invade the urinary tract. The main cause of the invasion is sex, which can push those bad bugs into your urethra and bladder, causing that burning sensation when you go to the loo (see What's Giving You A Pain? p.54). The more sex you have and the more vigorous it is, the greater the chance that bacteria will enter the urethra. Common symptoms include:

- Needing to pee every few minutes.
- Burning when you try to pee.
- Needing to pee with hardly anything coming out.

THINGS THAT CAN MAKE YOUR LOVE BOX REEK

- High-odour lifestyle, for example, lots of garlic or smoking.
- Tight clothing and synthetic underwear prevent air from circulating down there, creating a moist environment for bacteria to over-grow.
- Stress – it plays havoc with your hormones.
- Skipping your daily wash – make sure you swish plenty of water round those lips every day.
- Douching (see 6 Very Convincing Reasons To Douche No More p.44).
- Using feminine hygiene sprays. They mess with your vagina's perfect bacterial balance. Anything scented or deodorised is usually a bad idea down there.
- Listen to what your mum taught you: wipe properly front to back. Otherwise you're just smearing poo all over your joy hole.
- Forgotten items: diaphragm, tampon, sex toy, or salad item left inside, for instance.

- Some blood in your pee (pink pee).
- Pain just above your pubic bone.
- Strong odour to your morning's first pee.

You'll need to take antibiotics. UTIs can cause serious damage, including infertility, if left untreated. Ask your doctor for a two- or three-day course, which is as effective as the more common seven-day course and may reduce the risk of an antibiotics-related yeast infection like thrush.

Here's how you can stay healthy next time you have too much of a good thing:

- Make a bathroom run before and after sex, and wipe from front to back to keep nasty bacteria out of your urethra.
- Be extra vigilant before your period and during ovulation, when hormonal changes make it ideal for bacteria to grow.
- Drink plenty of water to flush out UTI-causing bacteria.
- If you're prone to UTIs, take cranberry capsules (more potent than juice). Cranberries contains proanthocyanidin chemicals, which prevent bacteria from attaching to your bladder wall.
- Antiseptics and perfumes can irritate the vulva and the opening of the urethra, and make the problem worse, so don't use antiseptic wipes, perfumed soap, antiseptics or bubble baths in the bathwater.
- Don't wear jeans that are too tight. The knot of seams can bruise the opening of the urethra.
- Friction, usually by the penis, seems to be a main cause of UTIs. A change of position may help as well as adding a dab of water-based lube, which greatly reduces friction.

6 Very Convincing Reasons To Douche No More

A vaginal douche is a process of rinsing or cleaning the vagina by forcing water or another solution (usually a water/vinegar mixture) into the vaginal cavity. Vaginal douches are available over the counter. There is a myth that douching after unprotected sex can prevent pregnancy but the opposite is actually true. If a women does douche after unprotected sex, it can push the sperm further up through the cervix.

1. Like the best ovens, the vagina is self-cleaning.
2. Douching washes away the good bacteria that keep your vagina's yeast population in check.
3. Douching can push bad bacteria into your uterus, increasing your risk of a serious infection, such as pelvic inflammatory disease (see Chapter Eight).
4. Douching can actually mean less enjoyable sex and less orgasms. Rearchers found that women who regularly cleansed their vaginal area with scented products ended up causing friction and damage to their vulva area, making sex uncomfortable.
5. Douching does not prevent pregnancy.
6. Douching has been linked with salpingitis – inflammation of the fallopian tubes.

THE BIG STINK

Ever since I started exercising, my vagina has been smelling funny.

Are you wearing stretchy workout clothes, along with synthetic underwear and tights? They are no friend to your love pouch – the material doesn't let air circulate. Result: a moist environment, ideal breeding ground for overgrowths of skin bacteria that, although normal, could be causing your potent bouquet. You may just be one of the women who needs to bathe twice a day, similar to men who have to shave twice a day.

> Bacterial vaginosis (BV) is not a sexually transmitted disease. You can get it even if you're in an exclusive relationship and you and your lover have always been scrupulous about using condoms. Always leave diagnosis to the professionals. Self-treating BV can be dangerous.

How come my new boyfriend says my vagina smells and tastes funny? I've had no complaints in the past.

There are conditions as simple as thrush and as serious as bacterial vaginosis (BV), which cause vaginal odour, but it sounds like the main condition you have comes attached with a penis. Women do have an odour. But then, so does chocolate, the ocean, green grass, bananas and just about everything else organic in the world – including men. And since his semen mingles with your own fluids during intercourse, it could be that what he is reacting to his own sweet smell!

I recently noticed a change in my vagina's smell. Not bad, just different.

The most common reason your scent changes is infection – the most likely culprits being thrush, trichomoniasis (see Chapter Eight), or bacterial vaginosis (BV) (see left). These are usually accompanied by a foul scent, which doesn't sound like what you are experiencing. Diet changes, hormone fluctuations linked to your menstrual cycle, pregancy or stress, contraceptives that contain hormones (the Pill, patches, implants, the ring), sexual arousal, a new sex partner or spermicide and vaginal infections can all give you a different eau de vagina.

My vagina smells fishy. Is this normal?

In spite of locker-room jokes, the vagina does not normally smell fishy. If yours pongs of something washed up on the beach, it is almost certain that you have bacterial vaginosis (BV), a bacterial infection that affects up to 30 per cent of women regularly. It also comes with a creamy white or greyish vaginal discharge and redness around the vagina.

6 Every Day Things That Can Make you Scratch

Bust these below-the-belt blunders before you start itching:

(1) Tight clothes: Peel-on jeans and tights can cause redness and irritation.

(2) Not lubing up: Vaginal dryness makes sex the equivalent of rubbing sandpaper on your delicate vaginal skin, causing rashes.

(3) Pantyliners: Friction from the liner can irritate delicate tissues. Use ultrathin pads when suitable.

(4) Disguising your scent: Scented soaps, talc, pantyliners and tampons have chemicals that can cause irritations.

(5) Getting too clean: This can irritate your vulva. There's no need to wash several times a day – once is usually sufficient.

(6) Not doing yoga: Being stressed or anxious can cause itching.

The Usual Itch Suspects

SUSPECT	WANTED FOR	KNOWN ACCOMPLICES
Candida albicans	Itching, soreness and/or cottage cheese-like discharge.	When something messes with the vaginal pH balance.
Allergies and sensitivities.	Mild to severe itching, burning, and/or red splotchy rash.	It's possible to have a reaction to almost any chemical substance that comes into contact with the vulva, from laundry detergents and fabric softeners to feminine hygiene products and spermicides.
Vulvodynia	Itching, pain	Unknown
Vulvar Intraepithelial Neoplasia (VIN), abnormal cells in the vulvar skin that occur in different stages of severity.	Mild to severe vulvar itching and burning.	Unknown, although it's been associated with sex.
Lichen Planus, a skin condition which causes inflammation and ulcer-like changes of the skin.	Itching, rashes, heavy, yellowish discharge, bleeding or pain with intercourse.	Unknown, though may be contagious and passed through sex.
Lichen Sclerosis, an extremely itchy skin condition which can occur on any part of the body including the vulva and anal area.	Severe itching, small cuts from constant scratching, pain during intercourse and flat rough white patches around the vulva.	Unknown, although it may be genetic.
Lichen simplex, a skin condition resulting from a chronic irritation. of the vulva.	Itching, burning, and/or thickened skin.	Allergies or sensitivities

WEAPONS (TREATMENT)	LEVEL OF DANGER (OTHER COMPLICATION)	PROTECTIVE MEASURES
Anti-fungal cream	Minimal as long as it's not misdiagnosed.	Try inserting yogurt that contains acidophilus (a live bacteria) directly into the vagina. Ask your doctor first.
Apply over-the-counter topical steroid ointment creams outside the vagina and take an oral antihistamine, both for one to two weeks until symptoms disappear.	Overuse of cream can cause thinning of the skin which will make your problem worse rather than helping it.	Figure out what's causing your irritation and steer clear of all perfumed products.
Anti-depressant drugs	Painful sex	Stress-relief techniques
If severe, the abnormal cells will be removed via laser or cutting out.	It can be a warning signal of a cancerous condition.	Keep your follow-up appointments to ensure the condition has not become cancerous.
Topical steroid ointment creams	see 6 Everyday Things That Can Make You Scratch on p.45	None
Topical steroid ointment creams. If symptoms do not improve with treatment, a biopsy or small skin sample may be taken to rule out other skin conditions.	If it isn't treated, the lips of the vulva eventually shrink, the vaginal opening narrows and sex becomes painful.	None
Identifying the irritant and using topical steroids to temporarily relieve symptoms.	As a result of constant vulvar scratching, the skin thickens, itches more, then is scratched again. Many doctors refer to this as an itch-scratch cycle.	Soak 2–3 times a day for 10–15 minutes in luke warm bath water with 4–5 tablespoons of baking soda to help soothe vulvar itching and burning.

The Usual Itch Suspects

SUSPECT	WANTED FOR	KNOWN ACCOMPLICES
Vulvar vestibulitis (see Pain Killers on p.53)	Itching, severe pain when any contact is made with the vagina.	Unknown
Trichomoniasis	Itching, foul-smelling discharge, soreness or pain. Men often don't have symptoms.	An organism that is sexually transmitted.
Psoriasis	Extreme itchiness (unlike psoriasis on other parts of the body, vulval psoriasis is usually smooth). You can have psoriasis on the vulva without having it anywhere else on your body.	Unknown, although it may be genetic. While stress can set it off, psoriasis can appear any time.
Atrophic Vaginitis	Itching, painful peeing and intercourse.	Oestrogen-deficiency, most commonly occurs in women who use progestin contraceptives, are menopausal, breastfeeding or have had their ovaries removed.
BV (see The Big Stink on p.44)	Itchiness, foamy, frothy and greyish discharge with an unpleasant, fishy odour.	Infected bacteria in the vulva region.

WEAPONS (TREATMENT)	LEVEL OF DANGER (OTHER COMPLICATION)	PROTECTIVE MEASURES
Lidocaine gel may be prescribed to numb the area before intercourse.	Painful sex	A and D Ointment, and witch hazel pads may soothe irritated skin.
Antibiotics	It can increase your risk of HIV.	Using condoms
There is no cure. Topical steroid cream can relieve the symptoms within two weeks.	see 6 Everyday Things That Can Make You Scratch on p.45	Practising stress-relief techniques
Oestrogen replacement therapy	You may need to take progesterone as well to create a hormonal balance.	Using lubricants with intercourse
Antibiotics	If untreated, it can lead to PID, increased risk of STDs, and pregnancy complication.	Keeping the area clean

All women have harmless bacteria in their vaginal passage. In BV, the good bacteria is reduced, allowing the bad guys – like gardnerella – to take over. Some researchers think that anything that changes the balance of bacteria in the vagina could make some women more likely to develop the infection. This might include:

- multiple sexual partners
- frequent douching
- antibiotics
- hormonal contraception
- IUDs
- diabetes
- the menopause

Treatment is a brief course of oral or topical antibiotics. Unfortunately, the cure may not be permanent. The symptoms return in about half of women. In this situation, see your doctor again for a repeat of treatment or to try another antibiotic.

DITCH THE ITCH

My vagina itches like crazy. Is it an infection?

It's not necessarily an infection. There are dozens of things that could cause an itchy vagina. It depends on what other symptoms you have.

The problem is when you think you know what it is, and grab some over-the-counter medication, you could make things worse. For instance, if you think it's thrush and start applying the antifungal cream, but it's really bacterial vaginosis, then you put yourself at risk of pelvic inflammatory disease (see Chapter Eight) and possibly, if left untreated, infertility. You may simply be having an allergic reaction to a new soap and slathering on the antifungal cream will play all sorts of havoc with your basically healthy vagina's natural balance.

About 1 woman in 5 has no thrush symptoms.

Just remember that there are many conditions that can cause genital itching and you're not qualified to guess which is causing yours. To get a low-down on your itch, see The Usual Itch Suspects on these and the previous pages and get it checked out by a doctor.

What's the difference between a yeast infection and thrush?

Nothing. They're both terms for candida – and to make things even more confusing, it's also known as candidiasis and monilial vaginitis.

Candida albicans (a fungus responsible for most vaginal yeast infections) lives quite happily in our bowels, vagina and on the skin and usually gives us no trouble. But if your immune system is down, the candida can go out of control – think of it as a teenager who realises her parents will be away for the weekend and she can throw a party. That's when it becomes candidiadis. You'll notice a whole round of unpleasant symptoms: white, cottage cheese-like discharge, painful urination, and intensely itchy genitals.

Could I have thrush and not know it?

Yes. But if you don't have any obvious symptoms, such as itching, burning and swelling, don't worry about it. Thrush in itself is not dangerous, even if left untreated. The problem is when another truly dangerous infection is misdiagnosed as thrush (see The Big Stink on p.44).

I seem to get thrush frequently. What's wrong?

The problem with yeast is it's ALIVE! And it's stubborn, smart and simple in its ambitions. Even if you treat your thrush with the proper medication, it doesn't clean the house completely. Tiny numbers of the yeast remain. If your defences are down, it starts growing again. But rather than a repeat performance of its last appearance, it undergoes a makeover, making the treatment less effective the next time you use it. The key is to switch medication if it seems that the yeast has second-guessed you.

You might consider taking 'suppressive' therapy. This usually means taking an anti-thrush tablet, prescribed by your doctor, every day or once a week (depending on which product it is). However, you may want to think twice about taking a prescription drug on a daily basis for a condition that is not seriously hazardous.

There are a couple of non-medical suggestions that many people swear helps their thrush. There is no scientific evidence that any of these have any effect, but they probably won't hurt either. Smearing bio ('live') yogurt over your vulva and inside your vagina may help keep a healthy vaginal environment. Put a dab of yogurt on a tampon and insert so the yogurt is pushed into the top of the vagina , then remove the tampon an hour later.

Another possibility is diluting 20 drops of tea tree oil in half a cup of water, soaking a tampon in this

Signs Of Thrush

You may have all, some or none of these if you have a thrush:

(1) Itching and/or burning.
(2) White, thick lumpy discharge (it looks like cottage cheese and may smell bad).
(3) Redness and swelling of the vulva.
(4) Painful sex.
(5) Pain or burning when peeing.

THRUSH CHECKS AND BALANCES

Answer yes to any of the following and you may be creating a breeding ground for thrush.

Are you a woman?
Oestrogen seems to play a role in triggering yeast growth. Many women are prone to the infections just before or after they menstruate and during pregnancy, most likely because of fluctuating hormone levels. Women on the Pill may also develop these infections. Switching to an oral contraceptive with less oestrogen can sometimes help.

Do you wear pantyliners?
Yeast organisms thrive in moist warm environments. Pantyliners, which are designed to absorb menstrual discharge, aren't 'porous' for the obvious reason. So unlike cotton pants, say, they don't 'breathe'.

Are you taking antibiotics?
Broad-spectrum antibiotics, including tetracycline and penicillin, can trigger a thrush by killing off 'good' bacteria that keep yeast in check.

Are you a lover of sweets, carbohydrates or alcohol?
Many people with recurring thrush find that there is a dramatic improvement when they stop eating foods containing significant amounts of sugar, fructose, and dextrose. Yeast thrives on these simple carbohydrates. Alcohol contains a high level of quick-acting carbohydrates. By drinking an alcoholic beverage, you may be feeding the yeast.

Are you a mermaid?
Don't sit around in a wet bathing suit. The chlorine in swimming pools can affect the vagina, leading to a chemical-induced irritation that may allow vaginal thrush to act up.

Are you into internal showers?
Douching removes the healthy secretions and dries the surface of the vagina. Normal bacteria are also washed away which allows for overgrowth of yeast.

Are you a germ phobe?
Antibacterial soaps are not a good idea as they may kill the good bugs.

Do you live in a hot climate?
Because thrush thrives in warm, moist environments, you are more prone to thrush when the temperature climbs.

Are you stressed?
Stress can trigger thrush. Physical and emotional stress may lower your resistance and predispose you to flare-ups, just as it can make you more prone to colds and herpes outbreaks.

Do you wear a tampon?
Deodorant tampons may irritate already inflamed skin and worsen symptoms. In addition, if you have some vaginal yeast, wearing super-absorbent tampons for long periods of time could aggravate an infection. Instead, try regular-absorbency cotton tampons.

Are you a back-wiper?
Doctors think that wiping from back-to-front as opposed to front-to-back may be how thrush gets started, because bacteria is introduced into the vagina.

Do you have diabetes?
Diabetes raises blood sugar levels, making the body a good environment for yeast to grow. Thrush may occur often and is harder to deal with when blood sugars are not under control.

CERVICITIS

If you experience pain during sex, with an accompanying discharge, you may have cervicitis, an inflammation of the cervix (the base of the uterus that opens into the back of the vagina). Cervicitis is most often caused by a sexually transmitted infection (such as herpes, gonorrhoea, trichomoniasis, or chlamydia – see Chapter Eight), but can also be caused by injury or trauma to the cervix, or from allergic reactions to certain chemicals that are placed in the vagina (including those in latex condoms, spermicides, tampons, or douches).

Cervicitis can be hard to diagnose because some women can have chronic (long-term) inflammation of their cervix, and experience no symptoms. In these cases, the infection is diagnosed by a gynaecologist. When there are symptoms, they can range from mild to severe, and can include:

● Vaginal discharge that may have a strong smell, contain pus, and/or become heavier right after menstruation.
● 'Spotting' between periods or after intercourse.
● Genital itching and burning, pelvic pain, and/or pain during intercourse.
● Painful, burning urination.
● Lower back pain.

Once cervicitis is diagnosed, treatment depends on the cause and how bad the infection is. Cervicitis caused by bacterial STIs (such as gonorrhoea) are usually treated with antibiotics or other medications.

If the inflammation is caused by an allergic reaction or irritation, you'll need to figure out the cause – douching, using scented soap or tampons, etc. Women who have chronic cervicitis might need surgery to remove any abnormal cell growth from the outer surface of the cervix, allowing new healthy tissue to grow in its place.

It is important to get cervicitis diagnosed in the early stages, because if left untreated, it can increase your risks of infertility and problems in pregnancy, including miscarriage and premature labour. Symptoms don't show, so regular check-ups are key.

---

liquid and then inserting it into the vagina. Change it as frequently as you would a normal tampon.

I've got thrush and it won't die. I've tried over-the-counter medication with no relief.

Your body may have become too used to the medication you are using. About 20 per cent of women will develop a resistance to thrush medications, especially if they are of the over-the-counter variety (which tend to be weaker than the prescribed kinds). Switching brands probably won't help, since most brands have similar active ingredients. See your doctor to find out what else is available. Make sure you really have thrush and not BV or Trich (see Chapter Eight).

My boyfriend says he can get thrush if I have it. Is that true?

Very rarely. It usually works the other way around. Candida can grow in a man's seminal vesicle (located near the prostate gland). If he has a reservoir of yeast – which can result from antibiotic treatment or diabetes – he can pass it on to his partner if he ejaculates into her. Because such men are symptom-free, a woman has no way of knowing that her partner

> Chronic pelvic pain – pain that has lasted at least six months – accounts for 10 to 15% of all visits to the gynaecologist and 15% of hysterectomies.

is the cause of her infection. So if you suffer from chronic or recurrent thrush that cannot be linked to a specific cause, ask your partner to be screened (his seminal fluid will be tested). If he is infected, he can be treated with oral antifungal drugs for two weeks; the doctor will then repeat the culture to determine whether the thrush has gone.

Occasionally a woman can pass a thrush on to her partner. The man will develop a red rash and itching on the penis. In these cases, a doctor will treat the infection with an antifungal cream. The infection usually clears up within four to five days.

> Research has found that raw carrots and tomatoes are rich in cancer-fighting antioxidants carotene and lycopene. A weekly dose of five raw carrots and a one-cup serving of tomato sauce (the most concentrated lycopene source) or other tomato products may help reduce your risk of ovarian cancer. Other antioxidant-rich foods identified in the research are spinach, yams, cantaloupe, corn, broccoli, and oranges. Getting more than 90 milligrams of vitamin C and more than 30 milligrams of vitamin E daily also reduces risk.

PAIN KILLERS

My whole pelvic area seems to spasm and I seem to be peeing all the time. My doctor says I'm fine but I don't feel fine.

What you're describing could be pelvic floor tension dysfunction or a spasm of your pelvic floor muscles. These muscles form a hammock, which makes up the bottom of your abdominal cavity and supports the bladder, uterus, vagina, and rectum. Symptoms can include:

● Pelvic pain
● Lots of trips to the loo
● Pain during intercourse
● Pressure or heaviness

Pelvic floor tension dysfunction is pretty common and, more importantly, it's easily treatable. There are two types: the first occurs when the muscles are out-of-shape and cannot support all your pelvic organs, and the second, pelvic floor tension myalgia, occurs when something puts the pelvic floor muscles out of balance and right into spasms. Pain from a bladder infection or even haemorrhoids, having one leg that's shorter than the other, or a lower-back problem can all affect how the pelvis works. Over time, the pelvic floor muscles go into overdrive to balance things out and at some point can go into a spasm.

Similar strategies for treating a back spasm are used to treat the pelvic muscles:

● Heat. Warm baths or a heating pad can help relax the muscles.

> Ovarian cancer is often confused as 'just a cyst' but any cyst that persists needs to be surgically removed.

● Muscle relaxants. If your symptoms are keeping you from your normal activities, muscle relaxants can help ease discomfort.

● Physical therapy. You'll retrain your muscles so they don't automatically go into spasm. Physical therapy can also help show if your pelvis is out of alignment, putting stress on the muscles.

My pelvic area hurts all the time, even during sex. What should I do?

Pelvic floor tension myalgia often goes undiagnosed or is mistakenly attributed to other conditions such as an overactive bladder or chronic cystitis. Here's a quick way to get it right: think of your pelvis as a clock. Twelve o'clock is where your pubic bone is, and six o'clock is where your rectum is. Everything on either side is basically muscle. When the muscles feel tense and pressing on them produces the same discomfort that you are complaining of, it's a good indication that the problem is pelvic floor tension myalgia.

Pelvic pain is serious business and can be associated with infertility, so it is important to treat the problem before it spirals out of control. Any and all of the most common gynaecological problems – uterine

What's Giving You Pain?

TYPE OF PAIN...	COULD BE:	HOW IT WORKS	HOW YOUR DOCTOR WILL FIGURE IT OUT	TREATMENT
Progressively worsening menstrual cramps, pain during sex, lower backache, constipation and painful bowel movements.	ENDOMETRIOSIS One of the most common causes of lower pelvic pain, believed to affect one of every seven women of child-bearing age (see Chapter Three).	The very same hormones that make women who we are – oestrogen and progesterone – can also cause endometriosis, when the lining of the uterus, normally shed during the menstrual cycle, grows outside the womb. The misplaced tissue can cause inflammation and pain that can be incapacitating.	Pelvic exam or laparoscopy	Doctors may first try to control endometriosis with low dose antidepressants, birth control pills or drugs called GnRH analogs. These agents block production of female hormones, disrupting the menstrual cycle. Steroids that suppress ovulation may also be used but there are side effects (weight gain and facial hair). Endometrial growths can be removed using laser treatment. In severe cases a hysterectomy is performed. If the ovaries are also removed, the patients are six times less likely to have pain return.

TYPE OF PAIN…	COULD BE:	HOW IT WORKS	HOW YOUR DOCTOR WILL FIGURE IT OUT	TREATMENT
In up to half of all cases, women have heavy, prolonged and painful menstrual bleeding, painful intercourse, intermittent spotting, frequent urination or constipation.	FIBROIDS A quarter of all women will get fibroids, usually between the age of 30 and 50.	Almost always benign, these masses of muscle tissue can quietly grow in your uterus for years without causing any problems.	Pelvic exam and an ultrasound.	At first, fibroids are shrunk with GnRH analogs. If the pain persists, the tumours can be removed through dilation and curettage (scraping of the uterus); hysteroscopic surgery (using a slim telescopic device through the vagina) or myomectomy (when tumours are removed through an incision). Fibroids regrow in about 15% of cases. Fibroids can also account for 30% of all hysterectomies.

What's Giving You Pain?

TYPE OF PAIN...	COULD BE:	HOW IT WORKS	HOW YOUR DOCTOR WILL FIGURE IT OUT	TREATMENT
The urge to urinate frequently, with urination sometimes accompanied by a burning sensation.	BLADDER INFECTION – one of the most common bladder complaints.	Bladder infection occurs when bacteria inflames the urinary tract, the bladder, and, in severe cases, the kidneys. Most bladder infections, often nicknamed honeymoonitis, result from bacteria entering the urethra and bladder during sex.	A urinalysis or culture taken by your doctor.	Antibiotics eliminate most bladder infections.
Severe pelvic pain, fever and other appendicitis-like symptoms, including vomiting and nausea.	PELVIC INFLAMMATORY DISEASE (see Chapter Eight).	Many women often get PID with an STD. The infection is actually often the first warning that a woman is suffering from a sexual infection such as gonorrhoea or chlamydia. The risk is low except for women who have multiple sex partners and don't use condoms.	A pelvic exam and ultrasound.	Antibiotics can cure this ailment and in rare cases surgery may be needed to remove the uterus, ovaries and fallopian tubes.

TYPE OF PAIN...	COULD BE:	HOW IT WORKS	HOW YOUR DOCTOR WILL FIGURE IT OUT	TREATMENT
At first no symptoms other than pregnancy may appear, but after a while, abnormal bleeding or spotting occurs, followed by lower abdominal cramping and sometimes severe pelvic pain.	ECTOPIC PREGNANCY (see Chapter Nine).	This can be life threatening because the embryo implants itself outside the uterus, usually in the fallopian tubes. It can also be incredibly painful.	A pregnancy test usually detects ectopic pregnancy, followed by blood tests for progesterone and beta hG (human chorionic gonadotrophin) – a hormone secreted by the foetus that rises in a normal pregnancy. An ultrasound can also confirm it.	Methotrexate, a chemotherapeutic agent given as a shot, may dissolve the foetus. Otherwise an incision is made in the fallopian tube to remove the pregnancy or laparoscopic surgery may be needed to remove the foetus.
Bloating, heartburn and a dull pain in the abdomen. In its advanced stages, the cancer causes cramping, fatigue, pronounced swelling and weight loss.	OVARIAN CANCER This is one of the rarest causes of pelvic pain, affecting less than 2% of women. Many fear the disease because it has a high mortality rate and rarely announces itself until after it's already spread.	An overgrowth of cells in the ovaries.	Early detection is key: 60 per cent of women with ovarian cancer are diagnosed at an advanced stage. Most cases are found with an ultrasound or a special blood test.	Surgery, chemotherapy and radiation are the most common treatment paths.

ARE WE IN VULVA TERRITORY?

There are two types of vulvodynia. Here are their character profiles:

Dysesthetic vulvodynia
Pain that is spread throughout the vulvar region. It can affect the *labia majora* and/or *labia minora*, the clitoris, perineum, *mons pubis* and/or inner thighs. The pain may be constant or irregular and is not necessarily caused by touch or pressure to the vulva.

Vulvar Vestibulitis Syndrome
Inflammation and/or irritation at specific points in the the area that surrounds the opening of the vagina. The syndrome usually comes on quite suddenly, and is most common in women in their twenties or thirties. It is very distressing because you experience extreme pain when your vaginal opening is touched in any way. So your sex life is probably zero and it can even prevent you using tampons, wearing jeans or riding a bike. In extreme circumstances, it can be difficult for a woman to walk or even sit. Sometimes women who have this condition may find small bumps or sores – the size of a grain of sand – beneath this area of skin.

4 Natural Ways To Get Relief

None of the things below mean you should rush to the shops and ignore your doctor when in pain. If surgery is needed, that's what's going to heal you:

① EAT IT
What you eat has a major effect of endometriosis and fibroids, because your diet, like these ailments, can alter oestrogen levels. Women who eat a low-fat, high-fibre diet excrete up to three times more oestrogen and have as much as 50 per cent lower blood levels of oestrogen. Oestrogen-absorbing fibre also eases the constipation and diarrhoea that often accompany pelvic pain.

② WORK IT
Exercise reduces stress, which in turn can alleviate cramps. Yoga also makes you more flexible and so can help relieve the lower back pain that many women with endometriosis and fibroids experience.

③ BREW IT
Yarrow is an anti-inflammatory herb that can ease discomfort – try it in tea.

④ BOOST IT
Using natural progesterone may help block the body's production of endometriosis and fibroid-exacerbating oestrogen. It's available in a cream or pill.

fibroids, endometriosis (see Chapter Three), scarring left by an STD – can cause pelvic pain. But there are also many non-gynaecological causes of pelvic pain, because so many organ systems share space in the abdomen. It may be a urinary disorder (see Drips and Leaks on p.41) or bowel problem, such as constant constipation, cysts on the ovaries or an injury from extreme sports.

Other possibilities include STDs like chlamydia and gonorrhoea, both of which can spread to the upper genital tract and cause PID. Pain may also be due to emotional distress. Studies have found a link between chronic pelvic pain and past history of sex abuse, rape and other trauma.

An often overlooked case of pain is pelvic congestion syndrome (see Chapter Five).

Then there's vulvodynia, not a condition, but rather a general term that defines pain throughout a woman's pelvic area. Sensations can range from stinging to stabbing and/or piercing pain. The pain may be constant or hit occasionally. It might stay primarily in one area or bomb your entire pelvic region.

While the cause of vulvodynia is unknown, there are a few theories. Some believe that it is caused by an allergic reaction to environmental irritants, a hypersensitivity to candida or other bacteria, or high levels of oxalate crystals in the urine. Other research suggests that women with vulvar vestibulitis (one type of vulvodynia – see Are We In Vulva Territory? p.58) tend to be oversensitive and worry about things that may never happen – i.e. their brain is over-alert to signals from the nerves of the vulval skin.

Hysterectomy is one cure for chronic pelvic pain, but if you are planning to get pregnant someday you will obviously need to find a less invasive way to manage your pain. One new recommendation is very low doses of antidepressant, which helps up to 70 per cent of women and explains why the other name for vulvodynia is 'depressed vagina'. It's not because your vagina has the blues (although, considering the symptoms of vulvodynia, it would be a miracle if it didn't) but because these drugs raise the brain's dopamine levels, interfering with the transmission of pain. Anti-convulsant medication can help raise a person's threshold of pain. Biofeedback, acupuncture and stress-relief techniques are also used to help relax the pelvic muscles.

THE BIG C

How would I know if I had ovarian cancer?
It's tough, because only 24 per cent of ovarian cancers are diagnosed before the cancer has spread outside the ovaries. But research shows that 93 per cent of women with the disease experienced at least one early symptom that was easy to dismiss or blame on something else. In short, ovarian cancer is not silent. The signs are subtle, but there are symptoms:
- Bloating, fullness or pressure in the abdomen
- Abdominal or lower back pain
- Lack of energy
- The need to pee a lot but you don't have a UTI
- Constipation
- Lack of appetite
- Diarrhoea
- Nausea

Is there any way of knowing if I might get cervical cancer?
Certain lifestyle factors put you at risk for cervical intraepithelial neoplasia (CIN), a virus resulting in abnormal cells:
- Having lots of different sexual partners
- You started having sex before age 16
- You've been with a high-risk lover (someone who has slept around a lot)

Cervical cancer almost never strikes out of the blue in women who have regular check-ups. Cervical screening every three years is believed to have reduced death from cervical cancer by 70%.

- You smoke (nicotine promotes the growth of CIN)
- You have HPV (see Chapter Eight).

CIN isn't cancer – it's more a smoke signal that cancer may be down the road. However, you may not need to worry. Most early CIN goes away without treatment. The deeper CIN is within the cervical lining, the more likely cancer will develop (it's divided into three stages, with CIN 3 being the most severe).

Treatment will reduce your odds of cancer. The abnormal cells may be taken out, removed with laser or frozen off.

5 Questions That Can Be Answered In One Word

(1) Will shaving pubic hair make it grow back thicker?
No.

(2) Will peeing right before and after sex stop you from getting pregnant or an STD?
No.

(3) Can I get an infection if I leave a tampon in longer than a few hours?
Yes.

(4) What's a good tip-off that you have a vaginal infection?
Fishy-smelling discharge.

(5) What is one of the worst things you can do to your vagina health-wise?
Douche.

How can having lots of lovers be a risk factor for cervical cancer?

Certain join-the-dots connections were made from various pieces of research. This does not mean the conclusions are set in stone. While some things are known to cause a health problem, e.g. smoking and emphysema, others types of behaviour are thought to have some effect on the development of a health problem, e.g. human papillomavirus (HPV) with cervical cancer (see Chapter Eight).

Here's the lowdown: a high percentage of women with abnormal cervical smears have also reported having had more than one sexual partner. HPV has been strongly associated with cervical cancer because a significant number of women with diagnosed cervical cancer also have HPV. The primary reason for citing multiple sex partners as a risk factor is that the more partners a woman has (or the more partners her partner has had), the higher her potential exposure risk to HPV, boosting her risk by association of cervical cancer. This does not mean, however, that someone with one partner cannot get cervical cancer – or HPV, for that matter.

My labia are a bit lumpy, should I go to the doctor?

Yes, if you discover new bumps and lumps anywhere. With the labia, you need to check that you don't have early signs of vulvar cancer.

Vulvar cancer is also more common in women who have had an STD (sexually transmitted disease), especially HPV and/or HIV/AIDS. Post-menopausal women are also at increased risk, as are those who have a history of other genital cancers, obesity, smoking, hypertension, and diabetes.

It's most often found on the labia minora or majora (the inner or outer lips of the vulva, respectively) or the clitoris. In early stages, cancerous growths on the vulva can appear as pink, red, or white bumps that look similar to warts or rough patches of skin. Other signs that need to be checked right away are:

- Growths on or near the opening of the vagina.
- Rashes, warts, or sores that won't heal.

- Unusual genital itching, burning, pain, bleeding, or discharge.
- Colour changes or irritation of the skin around the vagina that last longer than two weeks.

Early detection is key to survival for vulvar cancer. When detected in the early stages, before it has spread to the lymph nodes, the five-year survival rate is 90 per cent. Once the presence of vulvar cancer is confirmed by a biopsy (the removal and examination of a tiny piece of affected tissue), treatment options typically include surgical removal of the affected parts, and radiation and/or chemotherapy. If large amounts of the external genitalia need to be removed, reconstructive surgery can help to recreate or reshape the lips and other affected areas.

What's the difference between uterine cancer and endometrial cancer?

They're the same thing. Only ten per cent of the women who develop this cancer are still menstruating – it usually affects women after the menopause. In fact, the most common symptom of endometrial cancer is bleeding after menopause. For women who are still menstruating, increased menstrual flow and bleeding between periods may be the only symptoms (which also may be symptoms of other problems – see Chapter Three). Carrying extra pounds and/or having diabetes, high blood pressure and hormone imbalances seem to be associated with endometrial cancer, so controlling these things may stop the cancer from developing or spreading.

BOOKS

THE NO-HYSTERECTOMY OPTION: YOUR BODY-YOUR CHOICE
(John Wiley & Sons, 1997)
by Herbert A Goldfarb
This authoritative guide gives alternatives on how to avoid a hysterectomy operation. It includes state-of-the-art treatments and promising advances.

HYSTERECTOMY: WHAT IT IS AND HOW TO COPE WITH IT SUCCESSFULLY
(Sheldon Press, 2002)
by Suzie Hayman
Well-known journalist takes you through what happens and explains your options and alternatives.

WHAT YOUR DOCTOR MAY NOT TELL YOU ABOUT FIBROIDS: NEW TECHNIQUES AND THERAPIES, INCLUDING BREAKTHROUGH ALTERNATIVES TO HYSTERECTOMY
(Warner Books,)
by Scott Goodwin, David Drum and Michael Broder.
Two fibroid experts reveal the little-known facts about preventing and treating fibroid tumors – without surgery.

COMPLETE CANDIDA YEAST GUIDEBOOK
(Prima Publishing, 2000)
by Jeanne Marie Martin, Rona Zoltan MD
This book outlines natural cures to cure yourself. The authors also teach you how to prevent candida in the first place.

100 QUESTIONS & ANSWERS ABOUT OVARIAN CANCER
(Jones & Bartlett Publishers International, 2004)
by Don Dizon, Nadeem R. Abu-Rustum, Andrea M. Brown, and Andrea Gibbs Brown
The book is written by a gynecologic oncologist, a gyneacologic surgeon, and an ovarian cancer survivor.

IT'S ALWAYS SOMETHING
(Perennial, 2000)
by Gilda Radner
Radner was a successful comedian in the United States. Completed before her death from ovarian cancer, the book is her personal account of her struggle with ovarian cancer and her inspiring attempt to keep an upbeat attitude during her illness.

INFORMATION AND ADVICE

Amnesty International
www.amnesty.org
An excellent resource for information on female genital mutilation. Log on for advice on what you can do to stop the practice and details on how to receive a human rights package.

Brigham and Women's Hospital
www.fibroids.net
Extensive info available on fibroids available to the general public.

The Bladder Pain Syndrome Association (BPSA)
Email: membership@b-p-s-a.org.uk
Website: www.b-p-s-a.org.uk
A support group run by bladder pain sufferers.

The International Pelvic Pain Society
www.pelvicpain.org/embolotherapy.asp
Established in the United States for health professionals to show how to diagnosis and manage chronic pelvic

The Fibroid Place
http://thefibroidplace.com
Links you to everything you ever wanted to know about fibroids and didn't know who to ask.

Baymoon
www.baymoon.com
Links you to many useful vaginal cancer resources.

OncoLink
http://cancer.med.upenn.edu/
Founded by University of Pennsylvania specialists with a mission to help cancer patients, families, healthcare professionals and the general public get accurate cancer-related information at no charge.

Yeast Infection Resource
www.yeastinfectionresource.com

The National Vulvodynia Association (NVA)
www.nva.org
An educational, nonprofit organisation founded to sift through the info so you don't have to.

The Vulvar Pain Foundation
www.vulvarpainfoundation.org/
This international organisation's purposes are to give hope, support and reliable information

The Cystitus and Overactive Bladder Foundation (COB)
Email: info@cobfoundation.org
Supports and informs women all over the UK who have problems with these conditions.

CancerBACUP
www.cancerbacup.org.uk
Europe's leading cancer information service, with over 4,500 pages of up-to-date cancer information, practical advice and support for cancer patients, their families and carers.

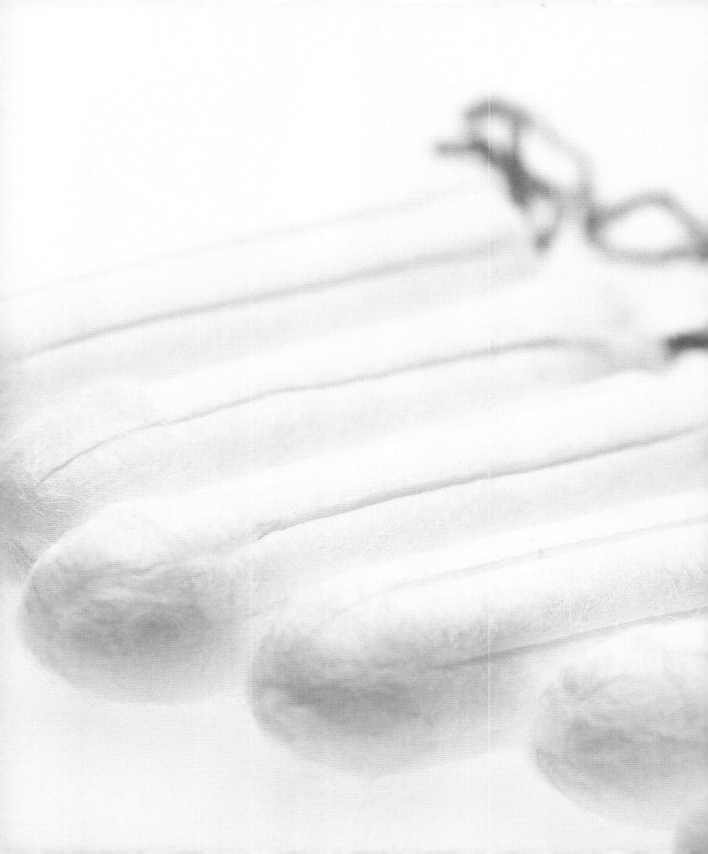

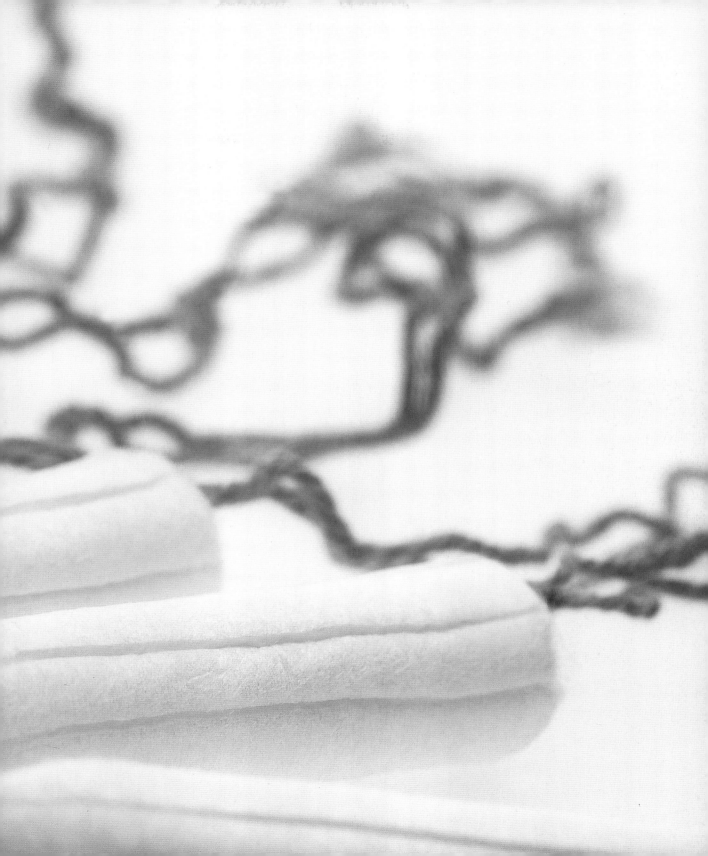

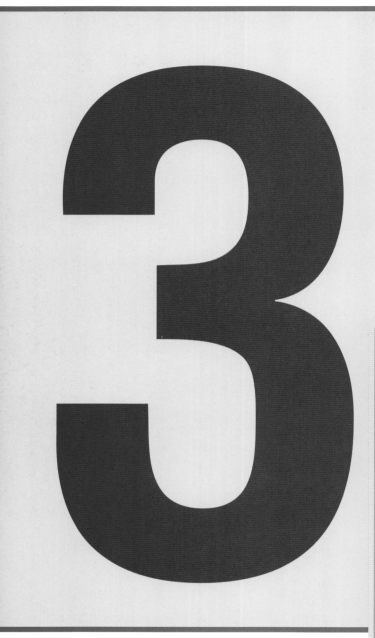

5 Healthy Cycle Habits

(1) An out-of-sync cycle isn't just a nuisance, it's a message about your health so get it checked out ASAP.

(2) If you have sex during your period, use lubrication – when you menstruate, your vagina actually dries out a little and friction can cause small tears in the vaginal walls.

(3) Also use condoms if you have sex when menstruating – your cervix is open and more susceptible to STDs.

(4) Build up your bones in your twenties with 1,000mg of calcium a day. By the time you hit your 30s, fluctuating oestrogen levels means bone density drops.

(5) Go on the Pill. When it comes to regulating an out-of-whack period, there's nothing like the oral contraceptive pill. With its timed release of the hormones oestrogen and progesterone, the Pill can bring just about any errant period into line.

GO WITH THE FLOW

Everything you do and don't want to know about your periods

Despite what you might think, your period doesn't just affect you when you're bleeding. In fact, your period is only one part of a complex hormonal, physiological and emotional cycle that occurs every month. On some level it affects you every single day. For instance, women who experience irregular periods and ovulation or show other symptoms of hormone imbalance may lose some of the protection that oestrogen and progesterone give. Their hair may become thinner. They may experience vaginal dryness, making sex painful. And, relative to other women of their age, they may be at a small but increased risk of early bone loss, which can lead to osteoporosis (fragile bones) before the age of 40.

Early muscle-mass loss may also be tied to irregular periods during your twenties. The problem is sometimes induced by extreme undereating or excessive exercise. Understanding how your cycle works – and how to work it – is a tool you can use to understand your sexuality, your body and your health. This Chapter covers everything you need to know about your fertility cycles and menstruation ('periods').

A MONTH IN YOUR LIFE

To get a better grip on what's going on with your body, here's a weekly guide to your 28-day (or so) wonder and how to work your hormones (everyone's cycle is slightly different, so the specific numbers are a guideline only).

DAYS 1–5: MENSTRUATION

The hormones oestrogen and progesterone have been steadily building in your bloodstream, but now they're beginning to take the plunge.
WORK IT: You might feel antisocial and lacklustre. Studies show you will have greater success in giving up smoking if you try now.

DAYS 6–13: PRE-OVULATION

Oestrogen is rising, making you feel perceptive and articulate.
WORK IT: Now is the time to schedule an interview or a blind date.

DAY 14: OVULATION

Oestrogen levels are still high. At this time, you may be beginning to retain water, but you'll still have plenty of energy. Just before ovulation, follicle stimulating hormone (FSH) and luteinizing hormone (LH) both peak. Studies have shown that high levels of FSH and LH can heighten your mental and emotional receptors, making you feel at your most creative and smart.
WORK IT: Your libido's raging, your body's primed to get pregnant and you're at your most man-magnetic. (Oestrogen can help to give your skin an extra glow. Your hair is also at its shiniest.) Recent research has pinpointed this time as your sexual prime, healthwise and orgasm-wise. Don't forget contraception.

DAYS 15–20: PRE-PMS

Progesterone, the nesting hormone, is turning you into a homebody. Now is the time to clean the house.
WORK IT: Elevated progesterone may also cause increased gum sensitivity, so avoid dental appointments at this time. Your appetite may be beginning to increase a little, as is your weight. On average, women temporarily gain about half a pound during this week of their cycle.

DAYS 21–28: PMS

The drop in progesterone can make you feel cranky. Oestrogen levels may cause the ducts in your breasts to dilate. In fact, your breasts may get a half-cup size bigger.
WORK IT: Think twice about all human contact – at least with humans you value.

PASS ME SWEETS (PMS)

What causes my back pain, body bloat, cravings and mood swings during PMS?

The theory is that your hormones are involved somehow. Possibly the fluctuations in the blood levels of oestrogen (which plummets) and progesterone (which surges) during the week before a woman's period begins in some way triggers premenstrual syndrome (PMS). But the truth is that no one really knows what causes PMS. So blame it on the moon, blame it on the economy, blame it on your cat.

If you are a drinker, be careful, as women tend to get drunk more easily during this phase.

   What is known for sure is that PMS causes a lot of women to suffer unpleasant side effects (see Blame It On PMS, opposite). Up to 85 per cent of women suffer from some degree of PMS, but only one in 20 are so severely affected that it interrupts their daily activities. It's usually at its worst during the seven days before your period starts, and it disappears when your period begins.

The Oestrogen Advantage

9 really amazing things oestrogen does for you:

1. Keeps your sex organs in shape.
2. Gives you breasts and other sexy curves.
3. Makes your skin soft and hair glossy.
4. Keeps your bones strong.
5. Acts as a brain booster.
6. Cranks your mood.
7. Perks up your immune system.
8. Stimulates the liver to produce HDL: the 'good' cholesterol.
9. Protects blood vessels (which may be why women tend to have a lower rate of heart disease than men).

Why do I want to eat a mountain of crisps before my period?

Your salt cravings are due to PMS. Other women have a weakness for sugar or carbs. In the last two weeks of your cycle, progesterone spikes, acting as a diuretic and causing you to secrete – and possibly crave – more sodium. Since serotonin (the feelgood hormone) also drops during this time, you may instinctively eat carbs and sugar to boost your mood.

If you can't fight your hunger, go ahead and give in – in moderation. Indulge in the one thing that will really satisfy instead of trying to eat around it. For example, rather than munch your way through an entire 1,200-calorie bag of crisps, satisfy the salt urge with one intensely salty and low-calorie pickle. If it's chocolate you desire, get a concentrated fix from a small piece of dark, rich chocolate. Bonus: Your body actually expends slightly more calories in the two weeks prior to your period (about 200 additional calories a day), so you can treat yourself to small snacks without piling on extra pounds and feeling guilty.

To help head off bingeing, munch on more whole grains, fruits and vegetables and eat smaller, more frequent meals. This keeps blood sugar on an even keel and wards off eating sprees.

I never had any symptoms of PMS before I turned 33, but now I have mood swings, food cravings and bloating. What's wrong?

Welcome to the wonderful world of PMS. While some 20-somethings suffer from severe premenstrual mood swings, the syndrome doesn't really hit until you're in your thirties. This may be because so many women go through a slew of physical changes at this time – for example, coming off the Pill to get pregnant, having a baby, stopping breastfeeding. You may begin to feel one or all of the following typical symptoms: cramps, cravings for carbs and/or chocolate, headaches, bloating, irritability, anxiety, impatience, and/or feeling generally out of control. In your thirties PMS can linger for longer. Instead of lasting the typical couple of days, it might hang around for five to ten days, making your life miserable.

BLAME IT ON PMS

All of the following have been identified as a symptom of premenstrual syndrome. Take your pick:

● swollen feet or hands ● bloated stomach ● tender, enlarged breasts ● weight gain ● cramps and lower abdominal pain ● joint pain ● skin rash, blemishes, or bruising ● headache ● nausea, vomiting, diarrhoea, constipation ● backache ● sinus headaches or drainage ● a sore throat ● changed eating habits, with cravings ● a cold or asthma ● irritability ● anger ● depression ● anxiety ● weepiness ● tension ● fatigue ● difficulty in concentrating ● nervousness.

WHO'S WHO

Your hormones are the movers and shakers of your physical and emotional health. Every time you get angry, become tired, laugh, cry, feel sexy, wake up, fall in love, feel so happy you could sing, burn with jealousy, feel hungry, or fall asleep, it's because your body is responding to signals from your hormones.

Here's how it works: the brain and body constantly chatter back and forth to sort of keep tabs on each other, alert each other of problems in their respective systems and maintain good relations. The vocabulary that they use is hormones and neurotransmitters (secreted by the nervous system). And the result of all that constant communication is the full range of human emotions.

Scientists have discovered that each hormone pretty much has its own distinct personality – some make you feel sexy, others make you want to spend the day in bed with the covers over your head. While they work together to create a balanced human being who can walk, talk and deal with life on a day-to-day basis, there are times when one hormone will seem to take control of your body and emotions. Just how much control hormones get depends on your menstrual cycle, your diet, your age, your sex, the weather, medications you may take, the amount you exercise, sleep and a million other things that effect the levels of hormone production.

There are hundreds of different hormones and neurotransmitters in your body, all doing their own thing. Here are some of the major players and their emotional effects:

DHEA

Whether you are male or female, there is more dehydroepiandrosterone (DHEA – easier to say) in your body than any other hormone. It bosses you around without reservation. Scientists call it the mother of all hormones because most of our other sex hormones are produced from it. It spurs your sex drive, your orgasms and your sex appeal, and generally seems to act as a mood-booster.

Oxytocin

This is a crucial bonding agent in relationships – a hormonal superglue. If someone holds your hand, your oxytocin level will rise. If that someone happens to be a person you like, just thinking about them will cause the oxytocin level in your bloodstream to go up. Actually touching will make it surge even higher. Curiously, it also makes you forgetful and diminishes your capacity to think and reason.

PEA

Also known as the love drug. When you are feeling happy, singing out loud, and head-over-heels in love, phenulethulamine (PEA) is probably at work. It has an amphetamine-like effect that makes you feel as though you are in a mind-altered state (it is also found in chocolate and diet soft drinks). Its similarity to diet pills is probably why some people lose their appetite when they fall in love. Low levels are believed to explain lovesickness. There is even a certain kind of depression caused by fluctuations in PEA.

Testosterone

This hormone maintains a healthy sex drive in both males and females. It is also your 'war-mone', triggering competitiveness, aggressiveness, anger and even violence when it surges. Which is why low levels of testosterone are linked to fatigue and depression.

Oestrogen

One of the female hormones (the other is progesterone – see below), oestrogen works overtime to regulate your menstrual cycle (linking it to mood swings), fuel your sexual drive, maintain your sexual organs, keep your bones strong, keep you safe from heart attacks, make you gorgeous (soft skin, glossy hair, curves) and regulate your fertility. When you're pregnant, oestrogen really flexes its muscles, getting you in shape for giving birth.

Progesterone

Oestrogen's buddy, this hormone also helps manage your period, sexual needs and sexual organs and preps your body during pregnancy. Progesterone also has a testosterone-like effect. It can make women irritable and aggressive – irritable towards men and aggressive in protecting their young. And whereas oestrogen stimulates cell growth, progesterone has a calming effect. For example, oestrogen causes the lining of the uterus to thicken and grow during the first two weeks of the menstrual cycle. Then progesterone kicks in, slowing the growth of the uterine lining and preparing it for the arrival of a fertilised egg.

Although oestrogen and progesterone reach peak levels when you're in your twenties, they give you long-term protective health advantages over the guys. His male sex hormones tend to cause trouble (makes them sound like teenagers). That trouble includes high blood pressure (which contributes to hearing loss), balding spots, and weight gain in the belly (which may mean future trouble with colon cancer). These problems are all deflected by female hormones.

Cortisol

This powerful hormone is designed to 'activate' your body in times of stress. You need cortisol to 'pump you up' to meet all the daily challenges of life. Without it you'd have no motivation to even get out of bed in the morning!

Serotonin

At high levels, serotonin promotes a sensitive side, a peaceful nature. That's why Prozac makes people feel so good – it boosts serotonin. But when serotonin levels are low, you may become violent, aggressive, and mean.

Vasopressin

This is the hormone that keeps your temperament from going to extremes. In the same respect, it may mute the intensity of certain feelings, making your emotional range somewhat narrower.

What Can I Do To Prevent PMS?

Because doctors don't know for sure what causes PMS, it's hard to know how to stop the madness. Start by experimenting with some of the many home remedies for PMS. Remember, what worked for your friend may not work for you, so you may have to try a few of the following things before you hit on something that works:

MILD TO MODERATE SYMPTOMS

PMS SOLUTION	RELIEVES	POSSIBLE SIDE EFFECTS
De-stress	Irritability, anxiety and cravings	A nicer, gentler you
1,200mg of calcium	Moodiness, cravings, bloating and pain after three months of continual use.	Stronger bones
50mg of vitamin B6	Anxiety and moodiness	Too much B6 can result in nerve damage – don't go higher than maximum recommended daily allowance (RDA).
Exercise	Mood swings, anger, irritability, cramps, headaches and lower-back pain.	A great body, but don't overdo it
Eliminate or reduce caffeine	Headaches, water retention, breast tenderness, anxiety and irritability.	Headache from caffeine withdrawal if done cold turkey.
Avoid alcohol	Depression	None
Reduce salt intake	Water retention, breast tenderness	None
Satisfy carb cravings	Anxiety, irritability, mood swings, mental fatigue, decreases depression.	None

SEVERE SYMPTOMS		
PMS SOLUTION	RELIEVES	POSSIBLE SIDE EFFECTS
Prozac	Depression	Nausea, dizziness, anxiety, insomnia, wild dreams, impaired memory and concentration.
Xanax	Anxiety	Drowsiness, addiction
Oral progesterone	Anxiety, water retention, irritability, mood swings	Drowsiness, dizziness
Diuretics	Bloating	Some kinds deplete potassium and have rebound effect of water retention when discontinued.
GnRH agonists	All symptoms	Infertility, hot flushes, lowered sex drive, bone loss, increaseD heart disease risk.

I know the symptoms of PMS but what I go through every month seems much worse.

You may be right. Doctors place the changes your body goes through around your period into four categories:

- Premenstrual Changes: Minor irritants like headache, fatigue, hunger, mood swings and increased sensitivity to pain.
- Premenstrual Syndrome (PMS): Symptoms happen together right around your period.
- Premenstrual Dysphoric Disorder (PMDD): Symptoms are so severe you can't function.
- Premenstrual Exacerbate: Chronic conditions you already have – migraines, allergies, chronic

depression and so on – get worse just before your period. Alcoholics drink more, smokers smoke more and bulimics binge and vomit more.

Diagnosis is through journal taking of your symptoms. If it turns out you're among the 5 to 10 per cent of women whose symptoms are extreme enough to qualify them for a PMDD diagnosis, the most complete relief may be provided by a serotonergic antidepressant, such as Prozac, Zoloft, Celexa or Sarafem (a repackaged version of Prozac approved specifically for PMDD). These medications can instantly ease PMDD symptoms, even when taken only during the two weeks prior to your period.

HOW WELL DO YOU KNOW
YOU PERIOD?

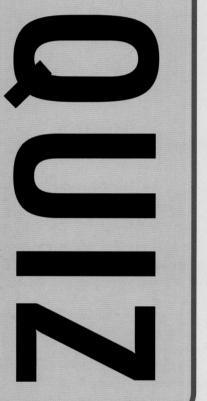

QUESTIONS

(1) When you have your period, you are apt to be:
a More irritable than usual
b Sleepier than usual
c Hungrier than usual
d All of the above
e None of the above

(2) To replace nutrients lost in menstrual flow, which supplements should you take?
a Calcium
b Iron
c Vitamin B6
d None of the above

(3) To find out when you're going to ovulate – and when you're due for your next period – count:
a From the first day of your period
b From the last day of your period

(4) Women who have very heavy or prolonged periods (for longer than a week) are likely to suffer from:
a Uterine cancer
b Anaemia
c Endometriosis
d All of the above

ANSWERS

1 (d) The production of ovarian steroids during a woman's cycles affects the centres in the brain that control mood and appetite, causing a variety of symptoms. The best way to cope is with regular exercise, sensible diet and more rest if your body craves it.

2 (d) You lose about a half cup of blood with each period – not enough to become deficient in iron or calcium, two minerals contained in the monthly flow. Taking a multivitamin supplement only during your period won't alter your risk for anaemia.

3 (a) The first day of your period is when your cycle officially begins, so start counting then.

4 (d) Because you're losing so much blood each month, the likelihood of anaemia is higher. What's more, research shows that women with heavy or prolonged (one week or more) periods are up to twice as likely to get endometriosis as other women. Heavy bleeding can be a precursor of uterine cancer later in life.

PMS OR PRE-M

Because the cause isn't known, PMS isn't easy to identify, since there is no specific biological or physiological thing doctors can look for. Diagnosis may take several months. Your doctor may ask you to keep a PMS journal and chart your symptoms to see if any appear consistently around the time of your period.

Some of the symptoms for PMS are similar to those for pre-menopause – basically, when menopause occurs before age 40. You stop ovulating and your periods stop completely years before the 'normal' age of menopause (51, on average). Be on the lookout for the following:

- Yul Brynner Syndrome: thinning hair is due to a shift in the body's balance of the hormones oestrogen and androgen.
- Extreme headaches, caused by perimenopausal hormonal fluctuations.
- Mad, Bad and Glad: mood swings are due to those pesky perimenopausal hormonal fluctuations.
- The urge to pee frequently: as menopause approaches, lack of oestrogen can cause the lining of the urethra, the outlet for the bladder, to become thin and less controllable, which results in the sudden need to urinate, even though the bladder may not be full.

- A need to count sheep, because during perimenopause, some women experience insomnia, especially if their hormone changes provoke uncomfortable hot flushes. Falling oestrogen levels may also cause difficulty falling asleep.
- Sex that makes you go Ouch! instead of Oh! – or no desire to have sex at all. Menopause doesn't have to kill sex, but changes in the vaginal lining brought on by falling oestrogen levels at menopause can make intercourse painful for some women. Others notice they have less sexual desire, possibly because pre-menopausal ovaries produce less of the hormone androgen.
- Vaginal Desert Syndrome: oestrogen decline can cause tissues of the vulva and the lining of the vagina to become thin, dry and less elastic, a condition known as atrophy.
- Night sweats: not due to the hot stud in bed next to you, but the result of sudden hormone-triggered changes in the hypothalamus, the body's 'thermostat' at the centre of the brain.
- A missed period: may happen as ovulation slows down. The time between periods will probably become more stretched out.

Period Protection
What works best for your lifestyle

SITUATION	TAMPONS	PADS	DISPOS-ABLE CUP	REUSABLE CUP	TINY VAGINAL LIP PAD
HEAVY PERIODS	*	*	*	*	*
ODOUR PROTECTION			*(because blood isn't exposed to oxygen)	*	
PHYSICAL ACTIVITY	*	Maybe (no water sports)	*	*	Maybe (no water sports)
ALLOWS SEX			*		
MAY CAUSE VAGINAL DRYNESS OR IRRITATION	*				
RISK OF TSS	*				Unknown
INCONSPICUOUS	*	Maybe, if small	*	*	*
EFFECTIVE IF YOU'VE GIVEN BIRTH	Maybe – if canal enlarged, it may leak.	*	*	*	*

Periodic Timeline

Add up the length of time you will spend menstruating between puberty and the menopause, and it comes out to about seven years. But every decade's period changes just enough to keep you on your toes when it comes to dealing with your 'monthly'. Here's how your age affects your period.

YOUR DECADE	GO WITH YOUR FLOW	BIGGEST PAIN	CALL THE DOCTOR NOW
TWENTIES	You're at prime baby-making age, which means your period comes like clockwork every 23–35 days. How your period is now is the baseline you'll use to deduce problems in the future.	Cramps (aka dysmenorrhea), which tend to be worse when you're younger or before you've had a baby (see Pain Killers on p.85).	If you're not pregnant and your cycle changes drastically (see Menstrual Mayhem on p.78)
THIRTIES	Your period may come more frequently, the bleeding may be heavier and last as much as seven days.	PMS comes to town. Your other problem: menorrhagia (see Menstrual Mayhem on p.78).	If you're leaking through your maxipad or super tampon in an hour or less.
FORTIES	It's anything goes: from total regularity to comes-and-goes as your body starts to run out of eggs. You're entering perimenopause, the 2–7 year prelude to the real thing (when your period has disappeared for a year).	You name it: irregular bleeding, skipped periods, early periods, late periods, or prolonged periods.	If you cramp or experience heavy bleeding. Either symptom may indicate the presence of fibroids, polyps, uterine cancer or endometriosis.

MENSTRUAL MAYHEM

Even the healthiest women experience occasional blips in their menstrual cycles, but how do you know whether to chalk them up to lunar shifts or to something more serious?

Here's a symptom-by-symptom guide to 29 things that can mess with your period...

The no-show period

WHAT'S NORMAL An occasional miss can happen.
WHAT'S NOT If you go two months or longer and you're not pregnant, you have 'amenhorrea'. The danger is that because your uterine lining isn't shedding every month, you may be storing up a dangerous supply of endometrial tissue (which can be a big problem for your reproductive system).
REASONS COULD BE...

- Diabetes: Treating the disease will often bring back your menstrual cycle.

- Childbirth and breastfeeding: These can also put a stop to your period for six months or more. Periods can also sometimes stop for a while after a termination.

- Ectopic pregnancy: This happens when a fertilised egg gets stuck in your fallopian tubes or ovary. Usually the only sign is a missed period, followed a couple of weeks later with pain in your abdomen and a small brown discharge, much lighter than your normal period. These pregnancies are not successful. The treatment is generally partial or total removal of the fallopian tube.

- Over-exercising: More than four hours a day, or running over ten miles a day – or too little food. You only have to be half a stone below your natural weight for periods to stop. This type of missed period is dangerous, because it's associated with a lack of oestrogen and that means a high risk of osteoporosis, not when you're older, but now. Even women in their twenties can suffer fractured bones. The Pill or oestrogen supplements can help restore normal periods and preserve bones, but if the condition goes untreated for too long, the damage may be irreversible.

- Drugs and medicines: Tranquilisers, antidepressants and medicines such as steroids or antibiotics can all temporarily stop your period as your body adjusts to the changes they induce.

- The Pill: If you recently stopped taking oral contraceptives, your body can take some time to adjust to secreting its own hormones that regulate ovulation and your period. The sudden halt in supplemental hormones could cause missed periods. Wait three months for your cycle to get back on track.

- Smoking: Recent studies show that smoking can cause skipped periods by lowering oestrogen levels. The cure? Kick the habit.

- Stress: If it strikes in the first half of your cycle, emotional upheaval or physical stress (such as an illness or travel across time zones) can inhibit the brain's hormone-sending signals. Wait a month for your body to readjust before seeing a doctor.

- Prolactin overload: A too-high level of prolactin (the hormone that controls the production of breast milk) caused by a non-cancerous pituitary tumour can halt ovulation (women with excess prolactin often start out with irregular periods, then stop menstruating). Other symptoms include headaches and a milky nipple discharge. Medication can control prolactin levels.

- Fertility problems: No period means no ovulation.

The overflow period

WHAT'S NORMAL Bleeding will usually fill a 50ml cup. That equals about a large tablespoon (it seems like more because it's mixed with water and other fluids).

WHAT'S NOT Bleeding 80ml of blood each month means you have menorrhagia (clue: you leak considerably during the night or you routinely start soaking through a maxi pad or a super tampon within an hour).

REASONS COULD BE…

- Miscarriage: If your flow is suddenly heavier and your period is later than usual, you may be having an early miscarriage (a whopping 60 per cent of all pregnancies end in miscarriage, the vast majority very early on – often before a woman even knows she is pregnant).
- Fibroids: They stretch the uterine lining and if there's more lining, there's more blood to lose. The result is heavier periods. You may also notice blood clots.
- Adenomyosis: Glandular tissue that's similar to the lining of the uterus is found in clusters inside the uterine wall, causing increased bleeding every month.
- Endometriosis: (see p.87)
- Polyps: Your chance of polyps rises steadily with age, peaking at age 50. Usually no big deal, these can show up on your uterus and/or cervix. However, if a polyp grows bigger, it can cause bleeding and cramping and, in some women, difficulty getting pregnant.
- Complications with an IUD
- Thyroid disorders: Eight times more common in women as men, thyroid disorders may, if unchecked, eventually result in life-threatening heartbeat irregularities. And if you become pregnant and have an untreated under-active thyroid, your baby's brain development could be impaired. Your doctor can prescribe medication to either replace or reduce the hormone; this should get your cycle back on track.
- Age: As you hit your mid-thirties, your hormone system will begin to misfire at times. Production of both oestrogen and progesterone starts to be less predictable, making your periods heavier.
- Von Willebrand disease: More than ten per cent of women with menorrhagia may have this inherited blood-clotting disorder. If you've always had heavy periods, if your gums bleed easily, and if you have experienced overly heavy bleeding after a minor injury or operation, you should be tested via a special blood test. For every woman diagnosed with Von Willebrand disease, another 50 have it. Many women with undiagnosed Von Willebrand disease develop anaemia and may resort to having a perfectly healthy uterus removed to solve the problem. But while hysterectomy ends the menstrual flow, these women are still vulnerable to dangerous bleeding if they are injured or undergo surgery.

The mini period

WHAT'S NORMAL Bleeding that lasts 4–6 days.

WHAT'S NOT Bleeding that lasts less than two days if you are not on hormonal contraceptives.

REASONS COULD BE…

- Thyroid disorders: see left
- Fertility problems: An extra-light flow usually means the uterine lining hasn't built up much and can simply signify that you haven't ovulated. If light periods become the norm, they could point to fertility problems.

Periods that take forever to come

WHAT'S NORMAL Up to 35 days between periods.

WHAT'S NOT A period that takes a few months to come signals oligomenorrhea.

REASONS COULD BE…

- Polycystic Ovary Syndrome (PCOS): This condition affects up to 15 per cent of reproductive-age women and occurs when the ovaries, which churn out all sorts of hormones, make far too little progesterone and too much testosterone, resulting in long gaps between periods, as wellas acne and noticeable facial hair. The real worry is that PCOS puts you at higher risk for uterine cancer (see Chapter Two), heart disease and diabetes. A doctor can prescribe oral contraceptives or progesterone to get your cycle back on track.
- Fertility Problems: (see The No-Show Period and The Mini Period on pp. 78 and 79).

Periods that never go away

WHAT'S NORMAL Some women spot when they're ovulating, around mid-cycle, because of a mild hormonal imbalance.

WHAT'S NOT If the bleeding doesn't occur at the same time each month or if it's less than two weeks from day one of your period to day one of your next period.

- Polyps: see The Overflow Period, p.79
- Fibroids: see The Overflow Period, p.79
- Endometriosis: see p.87
- The Pill Off-cycle: Bleeding may mean that your Pill's oestrogen content is too low (this is fairly common with some of the newer low-dose tablets). Ask your doctor to prescribe a different brand.
- A sexually transmitted infection: Chlamydia and gonorrhoea (both bacterial infections that are often symptomless in women) can cause breakthrough bleeding. Undiagnosed, chlamydia can result in Pelvic Inflammatory Disease and infertility. HPV may also cause bleeding after intercourse, which can be mistaken for spotting (see Chapter Eight).
- Early menopause: You'll want to know as soon as possible, so you can think about hormone replacement or natural alternatives, which may protect your heart and bones from the risks associated with too little oestrogen.

The moon cycle

The moon's cycle is the same number of days as the average menstrual cycle (the word 'menses' is related to the Latin word for months). Experiments have shown that women with irregular menstrual cycles have become more regular by sleeping with a soft light on in their rooms (to stand in for the light of a full moon) during the fourteenth, fifteenth and sixteenth days of their cycle, the days they would ideally be ovulating. After a few months, their cycles regulate. This is called the Dewan effect (although it may seem more like loony effect), and it seems to show a connection between light and the menstrual cycle.

IN THE PINK

Why do women menstruate?
In order to be able to get pregnant. The eggs that are fertilised by sperm and create a baby (or which, when unfertilised, bring on your period) are not created every month, but instead mature, one at a time, and alternate monthly in each ovary. That's why one month you can have a fairly mild period, but the next you can have painful cramps.

Your two ovaries act as a holding cell for your eggs. The eggs have been living there since before you were born. You started with one to two million of them, and by the time you hit puberty, you have squandered all but about three hundred to four hundred thousand of them through natural deterioration. These are the eggs that you have for the rest of your life.

Two hormones, the follicle-stimulating hormones (FSH) and the luteinising hormone (LH), are in charge of nannying the egg into maturity. At the same time, your body is pumping out more of the hormone oestrogen to make the uterus lining grow and thicken in preparation for the mature egg moving in. The egg is released into the fallopian tube. The fimbriae (on a diagram of your reproductive system, these are the octopus-like tentacles that appear to hold the ovary) help nudge the egg into the tube. The wall of the fallopian tube then has a series of contractions that move the egg towards the uterus (think of it as your fallopian tubes doing crunches).

A woman's 'fertile window' – six days during your menstrual cycle when intercourse can result in pregnancy – is extremely unpredictable. Only 30% of women ovulate according to medical guidelines – that is, between days 10 and 17 of their menstrual cycle. Which is even more reason to always stay safe.

4 Ways To Hold The Flow During Sex
1 Taking a bath right before having sex can slow up the blood flow.
2 Use a menstrual cup (see Period Protection on p.76) or diaphragm. Both work well to hold back menstrual blood during your period. (A diaphragm has the added plus of acting as birth control when combined with contraceptive jelly.)
3 If you use birth control pills as your contraception of choice, you can skip your period altogether.
4 Avoiding sex during your heavy days at the beginning of your period should keep the blood bath down.

At this time, another hormone, progesterone, is produced by the ovary. This is the nesting hormone, preparing the lining of your uterus to nourish and house an egg, should it be fertilised by sperm (it's also an optimistic hormone). If the egg is fertilised, even more progesterone is released in joyous celebration. If it is not, then the level of progesterone drops, and it is that drop that causes your period. In short, your monthly is basically progesterone blues.

If you're over 30 and suddenly start getting painful periods, get it checked out ASAP.

I think I've lost my tampon inside...
Don't panic. AWOL tampons are pretty common. It won't get lost in there forever. Even if the opening of your cervix is slightly dilated from childbirth, it's still only about as wide as a pencil. Most likely, the tampon's lodged near the back of your vaginal canal.

To find it, first wash your hands, then squat and fish around inside yourself with a few fingers (or ask your partner to do it). If you can feel the cotton or the string but can't get the tampon out, take a warm bath so your muscles relax. After the bath, try again to free the tampon. If that fails, call your doctor and arrange to go within the next few hours (don't worry, they've seen and heard it all and can get the thing out with a speculum in seconds).

Don't delay – a tampon left in for more than eight hours can cause a bacterial infection or toxic shock syndrome (TSS).

Is it okay to have sex when I have my period?

Sure. Just throw a towel under the two of you, so that you don't have to change the sheets (and this is not the time to break out those sexy satin sheets that cost a week's salary). Or clean the table, mop the floor etc, after sex.

You may even see more stars then usual: studies report that some women have better orgasms when they have sex during their period. However, even though your risks of becoming pregnant are low, they are not nonexistent. You should still ask him to slip on a condom if you both have not been given the STD all-clear, as the presence of blood can slightly increase the chance of transmitting certain STDs (see Chapter Eight). But if that's a concern (and isn't it always?) you should be using condoms anyway.

When is a woman most likely to get pregnant, before or after her period?

Before. There are three distinct phases in the average 28-day cycle: the follicular phase, ovulation, and the luteal phase. The first and last phases are mainly to prepare and create a comfortable environment, should she have received a visit from the stork. It is during the second phase, ovulation, that a woman is most fertile. It's the shortest phase of the three, generally occurring about halfway into the cycle (roughly 14 days before her period starts) and lasting for a couple days at most. This is when the ovary releases the egg into the uterus to lie in wait for a mini Gold Medallist to come butterflying in. The closer you have unprotected sex to that time, the more likely you are to be checking out maternity clothes.

> One problem with skipping your period is that you may not notice if something else is wrong. A weird period is one way to detect certain serious conditions, such as thyroid problems or uterine fibroids.

LIFE OF AN EGG

Women are born with a finite number of undeveloped eggs – around one to two million – in their ovaries. By the time you reach puberty and start menstruating, only about 300,000 immature egg cells, or follicles, remain. Some of these begin to develop with each monthly cycle, but during this time only one follicle matures into an ovum (egg) and bursts from an ovary into the fallopian tubes, initiating ovulation. Through a process known as atresia, many of the follicles that don't develop into mature egg cells deteriorate. As a result, only a few hundred remain at menopause, which usually begins at around 45 or 50 years of age. However, because of the hormonal changes that accompany menopause, the remaining follicles are unlikely to mature and become do-able eggs.

Can you get pregnant when you are having your period?

If you have very short cycles, it's possible. The maths goes like this: no matter how long your cycle is, you usually ovulate 14 days before your period begins. But the time between menstruation and ovulation varies a lot. For example, if you have a 28-day cycle, you ovulate on day 14 (28−14 = 14). But if your cycle lasts 21 days, you ovulate on day 7 (21−14 = 7). Thus if you have sex on the last day of a six-day period, you will have sperm inside you on the seventh day, when you ovulate, and you could conceive.

I stopped taking the Pill a month ago. Where's my period?

Hang on a bit. Depending upon the woman, the type of Pill, and the length of time you have been taking it, it may take weeks or several months before your ovaries are functioning the way they did before you took the Pill. In addition, if your periods were irregular before you started on the Pill, they may equally be irregular for a while after stopping.

If you have sex while you have a tampon in, could the tampon be pushed up to the point where you would not be able to feel it or remove it?

Your vagina is a closed pouch, but a tampon could get pushed up too high for you to retrieve it easily. You'd probably be able to feel it if you squatted and inserted a finger in your vagina.

Why does my stomach always get upset when I have my period?

Blame it on prostaglandins – the nasty little hormone-like substances that are secreted when your uterus sheds its lining. The prostaglandins make muscles in your abdomen contract, which in turn makes your stomach cramp and get upset. Try the following for immediate relief:

- Non-steroidal anti-inflammatory pain relievers or ibuprofen can block prostaglandins, not only easing cramps but also soothing an upset stomach. If your stomach usually gets irritated from aspirin, stick to ibuprofen. You should start taking them as soon as your flow starts so your body doesn't produce so much prostaglandin.
- Bring on the fibre during your period with whole grains, such as 100 per cent whole wheat bread or brown rice, and lots of veggies; hold off on extra salt, sugar, alcohol, spicy foods, and caffeine.
- Lastly, exercise usually helps keep your digestive system functioning smoothly. Although it's often the last thing you want to do while on your period, it consistently helps ease cramps and keeps your system on track.

How can I tell if my period is normal?

Forget using the 28-day cycle as a yardstick. Every woman's periods are different. Some last nine days, some three, others simply spot. The flow can be heavy or very light, dark red or dry and brown; clots may also be present. If your periods are consistent, then they're normal. It's only when your cycle changes in length or regularity or character – for instance, lasting only one day instead of the usual five or bleeding more or less than usual – that it's time to worry (see Menstrual Mayhem on p.78).

I have been bleeding after my period ends. Most of the time there is no pain. Sometimes I get cramps, however. What could be the cause of this?

Are you taking the Pill? Lots of women, especially those who've been taking the Pill for several years, experience breakthrough bleeding, in which small amounts of staining and sometimes cramps occur at various points in the cycle. While this isn't dangerous, you may wish to change Pill formulations.

Some women feel a slight pain or cramp during ovulation, some release a vaginal discharge that can include blood, some get headaches, gastric pain, and/or feel lethargic, and some women feel nothing at all.

Otherwise, you may have a vaginal infection (see Chapter Two), a hormonal imbalance, or a polyp or growth in or on the cervix (this last is especially likely if the bleeding only occurs after intercourse, see Chapter

> When women spend a lot of time together, their periods can synchronise with each other. It's thought to be due to chemicals called pheromones, which release each body's individual scent. Think of it as your bodies communicating with each other.

Your Cramp Decoder

Most cramps are the result of your menstrual cycle and are harmless. But sometimes that pain in your abdomen signifies something more.

THE CRAMP	OTHER SYMPTOMS	IT COULD BE...
Is a sharp pain in your mid- to lower back.	A burning sensation when you pee, blood in your urine, frequent urination and fever and chills.	A kidney infection which can follow an untreated bladder infection (see Chapter Two)
Gets worse when you have your period or after sex.	Very heavy, prolonged periods. You may also need to pee frequently or have constipation.	A fibroid (see Chapter Two).
Is in your side.	Usually nothing else but the cramping and pain get worse over time.	An ovarian cyst (see Chapter Two).
Is a dull ache between your belly button and the base of your breastbone.	Nausea and occasionally vomiting. Sometimes fever and pain between your shoulder blades.	An ulcer. A prescriptive antibiotic course can heal it in less than eight weeks.
Is a sharp steady pain under the right side of your rib cage.	Chills, sweating, fever and a loss of appetite.	Gallstones. If your symptoms are severe, go straight to the hospital. Otherwise, see your doctor for treatment.
Starts around your navel, then migrates to your lower right side.	Nausea or vomiting, fever, high pulse, loss of appetite, constipation, abdominal swelling.	Appendicitis. This is a medical emergency – head straight to hospital.

Two), endometriosis, uterine fibroids (see Chapter Two), or ovarian cysts (see Chapter Two). Spotting can also be due to an STI, such as chlamydia, gonorrhoea, or genital warts (see Chapter Eight). Excess boozing can wreak havoc with oestrogen, the female hormone that causes the lining of the uterus to thicken before it's shed during menstruation. Bottom line: if it happens more than once, get it checked out by a doctor ASAP.

I only have about four periods a year. Could I be infertile and not need contraception?

Don't chuck out the birth control yet. Oligomenorrhoea, when a woman has fewer than the normal 11–13 periods a year, doesn't automatically equal infertility. While you're almost definitely not ovulating when your period doesn't come, the chances are that you are ovulating just fine when you have a period (see Menstrual Mayhem on p.78).

How can I plan to get pregnant if my cycle is irregular?

There are a few different ways of trying to figure out when you're ovulating – unfortunately, none of them is foolproof. First, there's the time-honoured temperature method. This involves taking your temperature each morning before getting up or having anything to eat or drink (after ovulation there is usually a slight rise in temperature). However, some women who do not ovulate will still experience such a rise while others who do ovulate never have a noticeable temperature rise.

In any case, the best time for a woman to conceive is 12–48 hours before ovulation, rather than after.

You can also try examining cervical mucus, which

> Unless you are infertile, studies reveal that, on average, having sexual intercourse ten times a month leads to pregnancy after five months and having sex more than 15 times a month leads to pregnancy after three and a half months.

during ovulation is copious and can look like uncooked egg white, thickening up after the fertile period is over. However, discharge from any vaginal infection and semen will get in the way of your investigations. And not every woman experiences noticeable mucus changes.

Ovulation-predicting kits are now available from chemists. These measure the urine levels of the hormone that tells the ovary to release the egg and which increases the day before. However, most doctors give them the thumbs down. They measure the signal to the ovary to ovulate, but not whether the ovary responds. Some women have greatly fluctuating levels of the relevant hormone, giving false positive readings on the test.

> Orgasm may help ease menstrual cramps.

The best bet, and more enjoyable than any of the above, is to make love as often as you like, and not worry about timing it precisely to coincide with ovulation. You only need to time lovemaking loosely over the fertile period.

If I have periods does this definitely mean that I am ovulating?

No. You can have perfectly regular periods and still skip ovulation, which is why so many women do not discover they have fertility problems until they try to get pregnant. (Failure to ovulate accounts for 30 per cent of female infertility.)

Hormonal disturbances are usually to blame for lack of ovulation. Some signs to watch out for are the same as the ones you get when your period goes missing (see Menstrual Mayhem on p.78).

Light periods may also be a sign that you are not ovulating. And stress can often cause a hormone imbalance which leads to irregular bleeding, which in turn can affect ovulation.

Endometriosis can also cause irregular periods and infertility.

The only way to know if you are ovulating is to try to get pregnant. If you are still trying after a year without success, your doctor may decide it's time for further investigation (of course, you could be ovulating but your partner is shooting blanks, see Chapter Nine).

I've just moved in with my boyfriend. I know I'm not pregnant but my period didn't come last month.

For some reason that isn't yet fully understood, living conditions seem to affect women's periods. One study has shown that women who live in flats and hostels tend to ovulate less than women living with families and that students ovulate less than non-students. Women who move into shared accommodation will usually experience some initial menstrual irregularity and then end up menstruating around the same time.

Is there any way I can skip my period for one month?

Actually, there is no reason for you to have a period at all if you're not planning to get pregnant in the near future. Every month, fluctuating levels of oestrogen and progesterone prepare the uterus for potential pregnancy. A major dip occurs at the end of the third week of your cycle, which triggers menstruation. But if you try the following, your hormones stay steady so you won't bleed

> Nearly half of women with endometriosis have reported infertility problems.

(bonus: steady hormones also mean no PMS). And when you do have your period, it will be a normal one – not a build-up of all the ones you have skipped.

How can I cancel my period?

Try the following options:
- Seasonale: developed at the Eastern Virginia Medical School, this pill contains progestogen and oestrogen, the most common hormones currently used in oral contraceptives. You take it for 84 days consecutively and then skip a week, giving you exactly four periods a year
- 28-day oral contraceptive (OC) packs: when you reach the end of the active hormonal pills in a pack, begin the next set of active pills, skipping the week of inactive, placebo pills from the previous package.
- 21-day OC packs: instead of going through the pill-free week, start the next pack of active pills. Continued use of the active pills postpones menstruation by not allowing withdrawal from hormones. However, you may still get some spotting.

> Having orgasms and using tampons both seem to protect women from endometriosis because they prevent the back up of fluids in the uterus associated with the condition.

- Depo-provera: this is a progestogen-only form of contraception that's injected every three months. Good for women who can't go on OC, Depo-provera disrupts the menstrual cycle, tending to make a woman's periods less regular. For most women who use it, spotting between periods is fairly likely. Some women even stop having periods altogether.
- Hormone-laced IUDs: these also stop menstruation for some users.
- The weekly hormonal skin patch (and the hormone-emitting vaginal ring available in certain European countries and the USA) can possibly be used to skip menstruation.

PAIN KILLERS

I get killer cramps during my period. Is this normal?

Painful periods are not 'just part of being a woman'. So much attention has been focused on PMS that the pain many women experience during their periods seems to have been almost forgotten as a potentially dangerous condition. Dysmenorrhea – literally 'painful menstruation' – affects around 50 per cent of women to some degree and 10 per cent severely.

The culprit: an overproduction of pain-producing substances called prostaglandins, which are chemicals found in nearly every cell of the body. They regulate the tone of smooth muscles (the involuntary muscles of the body, such as blood vessels, uterus and intestines). An excessive amount of prostaglandins makes the uterus contract. In essence, the uterus squeezes so hard that it compresses the uterine blood vessels and cuts off the blood supply. This situation is similar to when the blood supply is cut off from the heart causing pain (angina). In both instances the result is the same: pain because the muscle does not have sufficient oxygen.

The pain can start a couple of days before a period, but usually it's most severe during the first two days of menstrual bleeding and then drops off. In addition, some of the excess prostaglandins escape from the uterus into the bloodstream where they may affect other smooth muscles. So prostaglandins are also to blame for the headaches, dizziness, back pain, tension, fatigue, hot and cold flashes, diarrhoea and nausea that can go with dysmenorrhea.

> Hysterectomy is considered a radical treatment for endometriosis and definitely not the treatment of choice for women who still want children. Also, the pain caused by endometriosis may recur following a hysterectomy.

Researchers don't know why some women have an overabundance of prostaglandins (although it may run in families), or why women tend to outgrow menstrual discomfort as they age or, sometimes, after a pregnancy. But prostaglandin-blocking drugs such as ibuprofen, a non-steroidal anti-inflammatory drug (NSAID), has been found to eliminate most menstrual cramping and pain and sometimes even prevent them altogether. The trick is to take the NSAID a few days before you expect your period. Continuously applying heat to the abdomen also relaxes the muscles and thus decreases pain.

What causes endometriosis?

Endometriosis is caused when some of the tissue which lines the uterus (the endometrium) begins to grow in another part of the body. Most of the time, this growth develops in the pelvic area – on the ovaries, the lining of the pelvic cavity, ligaments, or the fallopian tubes. Because these growths are made of endometrial tissue, they usually behave like the endometrium, responding to the hormones of the menstrual cycle. Each month, they build up tissue and slough it off. The result? Internal bleeding, inflammation, cysts, and scar tissue develop in the affected areas.

> Surgery to remove most of the endometrial patches followed by hormone treatment may be better at long-term easing of symptoms than just surgery alone.

Common symptoms of endometriosis include: extreme pelvic pain during menstruation; ovulation; excessive menstrual flow; exhaustion; lower back pain; infertility; or...no symptoms at all.

The latter is dangerous, because endometriosis can also cause other serious problems, such as ruptured ovarian cysts and an increased risk of ectopic pregnancy. The disease can be devastating and meddle with normal daily activities for days, weeks and even months at a time.

Before you ask, no-one knows why some women develop endometriosis and the type of treatment isn't even straightforward. Each case is dealt with differently, usually with a lot trial and error thrown in. The top theory these days is that endometriosis is caused by retrograde menstruation or a backflow of menstrual fluid. Largely made up of sloughed-off endometrial tissue, the fluid is thought to flow backward through the fallopian tubes and into the pelvic cavity, where the tissue implants itself and starts to grow. The research which launched this theory shows that many women do, in fact, experience this 'tissue back up'. This research also suggests that there's usually an immune and/or hormonal system problem in the first place that allows the tissue to take root and grow in those women who develop endometriosis. Although it doesn't set them off, endometriosis has been connected with certain cancers (think of endometriosis and cancer as two celebrities whose names are linked but no-one knows their real relationship): women with endometriosis are 30 per cent more likely to develop breast cancer, twice as likely to develop ovarian or non-Hodgkin's lymphoma, and 70 per cent more at risk for ovarian cancer.

Melanoma seems to be another risk.

> The most common symptom of endometriosis is pain. Some women describe the pain as sharp and burning. It may occur all month long, but worsens during menstruation, sexual penetration or bowel movements during menstruation. Women with endometriosis report wide variations in the degree of pain, from mild to completely debilitating. Many, however, report no pain at all.

Can having sex during your period give you endometriosis?

The truth is, no-one knows. The second part of the retrograde menstruation theory as the cause of endometriosis is that sex may push blood back into the tubes. But even if that does happen, lots of women have small amounts of a retrograde flow and don't develop endometriosis. Bottom line: it's probably safe to have safe sex whenever you feel like it.

Is endometriosis a cancer?

No. And it probably doesn't cause cancer. But certain underlying factors seem to contribute to both diseases:

- Both involve the abnormal growth and invasion of tissues. Endometriosis is a benign disease that acts like a cancer. Although it usually doesn't spread to other organs via the bloodstream the way cancer does, endometriosis can invade and destroy pelvic organs in much the same way.
- Both can be environmentally triggered; they have both have been linked to a pollutant called dioxin. Much of our exposure to this industrial by-product comes from food, mainly meats and dairy products. Dioxin stays in the body and acts as an immune suppressant and carcinogen. For instance, dioxin is known to interfere with the body's normal control system of uterine tissue so that stray patches of endometrial cells outside the uterus seem able to take hold and grow when they would normally be stopped.
- Both share the ability to produce new blood vessels.

5 Questions That Can Be Answered In One Word

1) **What puts you at highest risk for endometriosis?**
Menstruating

2) **If you menstruate early, does that mean you will have the menopause early?**
No

3) **What's the best non-drug way to keep PMS at bay?**
Exercise

4) **What's the best way to maintain your cycle and keep fertility primed?**
Sex

5) **Is it okay to miss a period?**
Yes

Cancer and endometriosis require new blood vessels to supply and nourish their growth.

- Both involve breakdowns in the immune system. Ultimately, though, cancers are an immunological disease, when the natural surveillance system that detects and destroys abnormal cells isn't working. Endometriosis possibly occurs because an out-of-whack immune system allows tissue cell overgrowth.

Is there a preferred treatment for endometriosis?

In about 3 in 10 cases, endometriosis clears and symptoms disappear without any treatment.

If pain is your biggest endometrial complaint, then your top-dog options basically involve painkillers:

- Paracetamol taken during periods may be all that you need if symptoms are mild.
- Anti-inflammatory painkillers (ibuprofen, diclofenac, naproxen, etc) may be better than paracetamol. However, some people get indigestion or other side effects with anti-inflammatories.
- Codeine alone, or in combination with paracetamol, is a more powerful painkiller. It may be an option if anti-inflammatories don't suit. Constipation is a common side effect from codeine.

To ease pain during periods, take painkillers regularly throughout of your period rather than 'now and then'. You can take them in addition to other treatments.

The next stage is hormonal treatments. Endometrial cells – normal or abnormal – need oestrogen to grow and survive. Reducing the amount of oestrogen that you make or blocking the effect of oestrogen on the endometrial cells can starve them of oestrogen. Therefore, patches of endometriosis gradually shrink, and may clear away.

There are five different hormone options. All have similar records at easing symptoms, but you can try a different option if one doesn't work (it may take a few months of hormone treatment to get the full benefit):

- The combined oral contraceptive pill is not strictly licensed for the treatment of endometriosis, but many women report improved symptoms when they are on the Pill (see Chapter Seven). The Pill stops ovulation, which reduces the amount of oestrogen made by the ovaries. Periods are lighter, less painful, and are predictable. Other symptoms such as painful sex and pain in the pelvic area may also improve.

- Progestogen hormone tablets reduce the effect of oestrogen on the endometrial cells, which causes the cells to 'shrink'. Progestogens also prevent ovulation, which lowers the oestrogen level. A Depo-provera injection every three months could do the trick (see Chapter Eight). Possible side effects include: irregular menstrual bleeding, weight gain, mood changes, and bloating. This is the only hormonal option that can be taken indefinitely.

- Danazol works mainly by reducing the amount of gonadotrophins that you make. This has a 'knock-on' effect of reducing the amount of oestrogen that you make. Possible side effects include: weight gain, hair growth, acne, and mood changes. On rare occasions, it causes a deepening of the voice that may be irreversible. It usually stops periods too. Treatment is recommended for six months at the most.

- Gestrinone is similar to danazol, but you only need to take it twice a week rather than daily. Again, treatment is limited to six months.

- Different types of gonadotrophin-releasing hormone (GnRH) analog drugs will stop the pain, as will menstruation – by throwing your body into a medical menopause. These drugs come in a spray, injection or implant form. A six-month course is usual. Naturally, this means you need to worry about all the other problems associated with menopause. Periods usually stop too. An option is to take a small dose of oestrogen and progestogen as hormone replacement therapy (HRT) to stop these side effects. This 'add-back' HRT does not affect the effectiveness of the treatment.

Sometimes surgery is advised to remove some of the larger patches of endometriosis. This may ease symptoms and increase the chance of pregnancy if infertility is a problem.

BOOKS

THE CURSE: A CULTURAL HISTORY OF
MENSTRUATION
(Dutton, 1976)
by Janice Delaney, Mary Jane Lupton and
Emily Toth
A fascinating read for anyone who has ever been
interested in how the role of menstruation and
repoductive capability effects social structures
and political equality movements.

PMS: SOLVING THE PUZZLE: SIXTEEN
CAUSES OF PMS & WHAT TO DO ABOUT IT
(Chicago Spectrum Press, 1995)
by Linaya Hahb
This self-help guide helps women to identify the
problems causing PMS. Over sixteen different
causes are identified here, with different
treatment recommendations.

TAKING BACK THE MONTH: A
PERSONALIZED SOLUTION FOR
MANAGING PMS AND ENHANCING YOUR
HEALTH
(Penguin Putnam, 2002)
by Diana Taylor and Stacey Colino
An excellent research-based guide to managing
PMS. It covers every possible scenario with each
chapter relating to your specific interest.

NO MORE PMS!: BEAT PMS WITH THE
MEDICALLY PROVEN WOMEN'S
NUTRITIONAL ADVISORY SERVICE
PROGRAMME
(Vermilion, 1997)
Maryon Stewart, Guy Abraham and Alan Stewart
The UK-based WNAS offer dietary advice and
eating plans to overcome symptoms of PMS.

THE WISE WOUND: MENSTRUATION AND
EVERY WOMAN
(Paladin Books, 1986)
Penelope Shuttle, Peter Redgrove
A classic, still in print after 20 years, this book
celebrates the creative strength and female
power of menstruation. The positive side of
the curse!

INFORMATION AND ADVICE

Endometriosis.org
www.endometriosis.org.uk
On-line support group.

The Endometriosis Association
www.endometriosisassn.org/
Offers a wide scope of information a few
different languages.

Red Spot
www.onewoman.com/redspot/
All about periods — a virtual gathering place
for the knowledge and experience that women
gain about their cycle over time.

Menstruation Museum
www.mum.org/
Check in to find out the rich history of
menstruation.

www.healthinsite.gov.au/topics/Menstruation_Dis
orders
For a comprehensive listing of menstrual
disorders, log onto to this site.

Many Moons
pacificcoast.net/~manymoons/index.html
Has been offering women alternative
menstruation products since 1989.

The National Endometriosis Society
www.endo.org.uk/
Offers information and links to local groups all
over the UK.

www.healthinsite.gov.au/topics/Menstruation_Dis
orders
For a comprehensive listing of menstrual
disorders, log onto this website.

www.theclothresource.co.uk/
Reusable menstrual wear means you protect the
environment, save money with funky sanpro! For
a long list of alternatives to throw-away towels
and tampons, see the resources here on this
website.

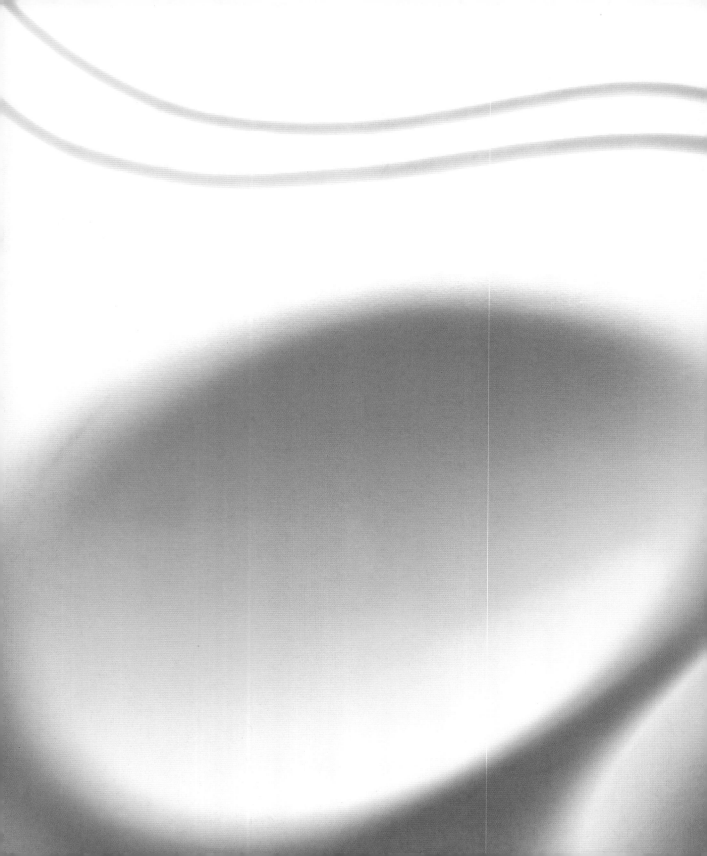

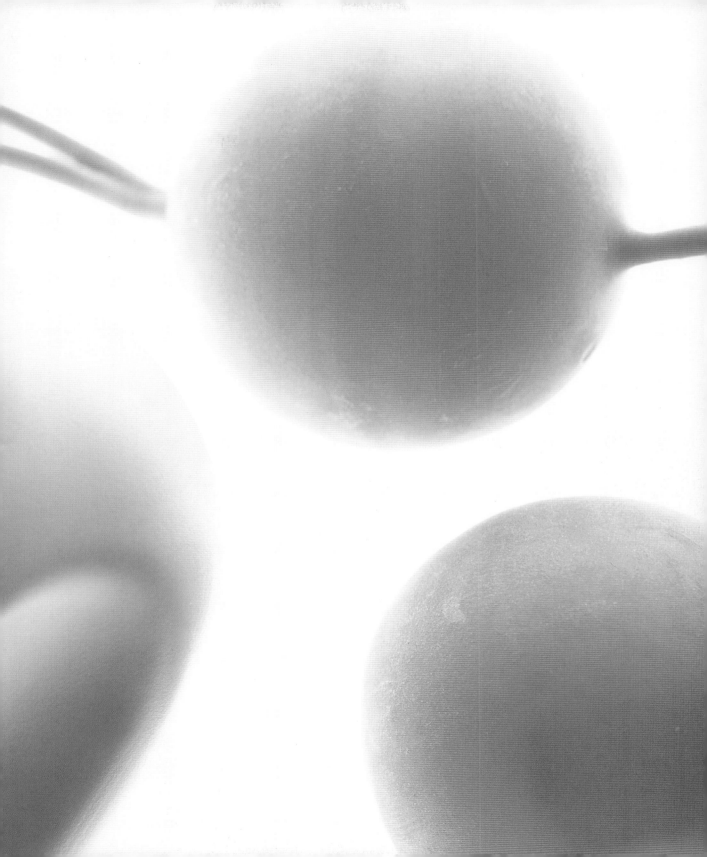

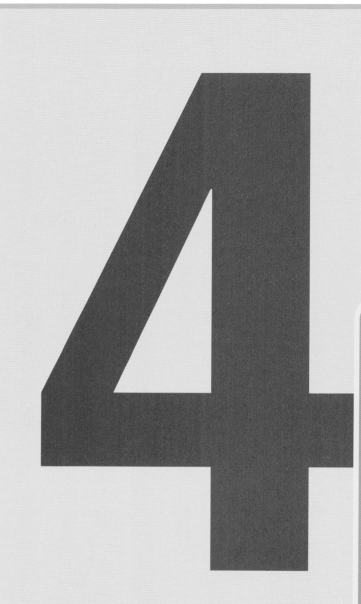

5 Healthy Orgasm Habits

① Get sweaty: regular heart-pumping exercises improves blood flow which boosts sexual arousal.

② Quit smoking: the nicotine and other chemicals in cigarettes constrict capillaries and choke off pelvic blood.

③ Do it lots: if you start making love more often, the chemical communication between brain cells quickens and intensifies because the impulses are travelling on a well-beaten path. The payoff is more orgasms with less effort.

④ Don't make faking a habit: sometimes it is easier to put in a performance. But every time means something is wrong and it's time to figure out what that is.

⑤ Lubricate, lubricate, lubricate. It makes sex more pleasurable and prevents painful (and potentially infecting) tears and cuts.

PLEASURE PRINCIPLES

Everything you need to know about orgasms

Surveys have found that as much as 70 per cent of sexually active women have trouble experiencing orgasms with their partners – or even by their own hands. Either they've never climaxed or they can only do so now and then or with effort.

The male package is no more reliable. At some point in his life, a man is going to experience all of the following: premature ejaculation, impotence, a loss of desire and painful sex.

KEEP ON COMING

Is orgasm really so important? Yes! Yes! Yes! Climax promotes cardiovascular conditioning, imparts a healthy glow to the skin, and improves overall body tone. In addition, the psychological benefits are very real. Because climax is experienced in the part of the brain that rules the emotions, sexual release decreases irritability and leaves you with a sense of wellbeing and a general feeling of relaxation. Some sex therapists even recommend masturbation as a cure for insomnia. And many women report that orgasm relieves menstrual cramps and headaches. So here's how to make sure you keep on coming.

Being aware of what goes on in your body at the climactic moment could help you figure out what's wrong when the earth doesn't move (not to mention give you more and better orgasms). So here's the action, play-by-play.

- Excitement: your orgasm starts before foreplay even starts. As oestrogen and progesterone production goes into overtime, you experience heightened awareness (this can also work against you – one false move by you or your lover and your whole response system can shut down). Meanwhile, your hypothalamus, the structure that keeps communication going between your body and brain, orders up chemicals to make you even more sensitive to his touch. As the physical action between you speeds up, blood rushes to your pelvic area (called vasocongestion), causing your clitoris to enlarge, your vaginal lips to swell and spread apart, your nipples to become erect and your breasts to enlarge by as much as 25 per cent.
- Plateau: the next stage is reached when your clitoris, now totally engorged, becomes hidden under the clitoral hood to protect itself from further direct stimulation. Meanwhile, your inner vagina expands as the uterus rises higher. Your outer vagina also swells and your vaginal opening decreases. This 'tightening down' can make it seem slightly difficult for a penis to get past, causing some women to worry they're not turned on enough to have sex. In fact, the complete opposite is true – the biological idea is to increase accessibility for the penis and vaginal stimulation for you. At the height of arousal, blood pressure doubles, heart rate can increase to 180 beats per minute and your skin becomes flushed.

- Finally, orgasm: with continued stimulation, the tension, swelling and lubricating increase until your body peaks and you orgasm – which, for all the hoo-hah surrounding it, is simply a reversal of the process just described. The blood that's been swelling everything like crazy is suddenly released and flows back to the rest of the body, the uterus or pelvic muscles may contract anywhere from 6 to 23 times (although you may not feel them) and the tension that tightens every muscle so marvellously suddenly relaxes as well.
In contrast to the earlier stages – which can last minutes or even hours – the female orgasm is 19 to 28 seconds long with an average of 23 (the male climax lasts only a few seconds).
- Resolution: this is the last stage. The body returns to its former unaroused state. Some people also develop a profuse sweating reaction, as though they've just finished a workout (which in fact they have). However, if stimulation continues at this point, a woman can re-enter plateau stage and have another orgasm. . . and another. . . and so on. It sounds easy enough, but the truth is that climaxing depends on every step in the process coming together. Result: orgasms don't happen every time.

DO YOU KNOW WHAT YOUR
(SEX) PROBLEM IS?

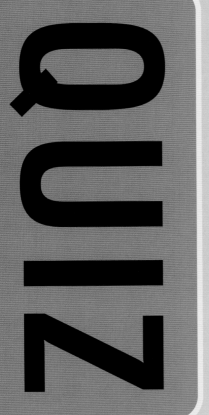

QUESTIONS

① **Women experience two physiologically distinct kinds of orgasm – clitoral and vaginal. True or False?**

② **How many consecutive orgasms can a woman have?**
a 2
b 5
c 25
d 50

③ **Arousal ends with orgasm. True or false?**

④ **How many orgasms can a man have in one go?**
a one
b more than one

⑤ **Put the following erogenous zones in the order they can be found in a woman's body, starting from the most external:**
a AFE Zone
b Cervix
c Clitoris
d G-spot

ANSWERS

1 False. The actual orgasm is the same whether the stimulation comes from the clitoris or the vagina.

2 (d) If the stimulation continues and she has the stamina, she can keep on coming.

3 False. Arousal is divided into four stages: excitement, plateau, orgasm and last, resolution – when your body goes back to its normal unsexed-up state.

4 (b) Orgasm and ejaculation are not the same thing for a man and if he can learn to separate them, he can become multiorgasmic.

5 c, d, a, b

ENTERING YOUR E ZONE

Is there really a G-spot?

Yes. However, just because it exists doesn't mean it works for you. Just like some women love having their breasts caressed others get off on having their G-spot pressed while the same pressing leaves other women yawning.

Whenever my G-spot is stimulated, I immediately need to pee. Is this supposed to happen?

First, make sure your 'urine' isn't really ejaculation. If it is urine, it will smell like it. If so, then your problem may have a medical basis: you may have formed an urethrocele, which is an out-pouching of the urethra. An urethrocele will leak urine when it's compressed, and that could account for your current urge (it could be worse – the pudendal nerve is also attached to the rectum). A surgical procedure called colporrhaphy can be performed to tighten the vaginal wall and provide the urethra with better support, putting an end to your wee problem.

SOLO SEX

Can you masturbate too much?

If you mean so much so that you're not doing anything else except masturbating, sure. But you can't get addicted to masturbation to the point where you won't feel like doing it with anyone else or it spoils you for intercourse. Orgasms are not finite – you can have as many as you want or need. Even men – who often need some rest time between ejaculations to recover their erection – can have more than one orgasm a day.

> 80% of men and 60% of women report masturbating regularly – and the rest are probably lying.

LET YOUR FINGERS DO THE WALKING FOR YOUR HEALTH...

- You'll get a clear understanding of your own anatomy and sexual response which means you'll be aware when something is wrong.
- It is the ultimate in safe sex – no fear of pregnancy or STDs.
- It burns off stress and anxiety.
- You'll be hornier – one study found that masturbators have more sexual desire than non-masturbators.
- You'll have more orgasms – according to research, the more you masturbate, the more easily you orgasm alone or with a partner.
- It keeps your vagina healthy by keeping blood flowing in the pelvic region.

In fact, research suggests that the more orgasms you have by any means, the more ready for sex you'll be. Orgasm – in both men and women – tones the pelvic muscles and keeps the genital area primed for response.

How come I always have an orgasm when I masturbate but never have one with a man?

This gratification gap is quite common. In survey after survey, women report that solo orgasms are more intense and speedier. When you masturbate, you know the exact pleasure pace and touch you like. Also, alone, you tend to lose your inhibitions.

When a woman's orgasm fizzles during sex, it's often because she's failed to concentrate on her own sensations. No matter how excited you are at the start, if you get distracted – say, by work worries or concern about how you look – the brain can override

Your orgasmic gush could also be female ejaculate, the other fluid women sometimes release during orgasm. You can tell the difference because female ejaculate is clear and odourless.

your body's responses and short-circuit the climax.

Banishing these pleasure-zappers isn't easy, but it is possible. The most important thing is to show your lover how to touch you the way you touch yourself.

You don't have to be a drill sergeant, shouting, 'Right! No, wait! Left!' instructions. Just take his hand and put it where you put your own, then move it like you move your own. If he's open to listening to you, you may be swept away by an orgasm as enjoyable as the do-it-yourself kind.

TURN THE KNOB

Can too much handling make my clitoris numb?

Rub your finger for five minutes every day for one week. Does it hurt after a while? Well, your finger doesn't contain a quarter of the nerve endings that your clitoris does. If your love button starts feeling like it's being anaesthetised, it's time to regroup. Soreness in the clitoral area is like a sore anywhere in the vaginal region – if the irritant continues, it can lead to infection.

Seeing a woman touch herself is often cited when men are surveyed about their favourite sexual fantasy.

I know most women can't orgasm unless their clitoris is touched, but I seem to get little pleasure from mine. What's wrong?

Nothing. Sex is like trying on a bathing suit – what works for one size won't necessarily work for another. Some women go wild when their clitoris is touched. Others would just as soon skip over that part of their anatomy, thank you very much.

9 Useful Facts About The Clitoris

(1) The clitoris and the penis are biological siblings. Both are covered with a hood, or foreskin, and both become swollen with blood during arousal.

(2) The clitoris is only the tip of a much larger internal structure, consisting of an impressive network of nerves, muscles and ligaments (see Chapter Two). During arousal, the whole structure swells.

(3) During sleep, the clitoris appears to gain and lose an erection about every 90 minutes, just as the penis does.

(4) However, while the penis has a couple of purposes: urination, ejaculation and sexual pleasure, the clitoris seems to have only one purpose: to give pleasure.

(5) Whether a clitoris is large or small – and there is a great deal of variation – bears no relation to sexual performance or enjoyment.

(6) What matters is the density of nerve endings in and near the clitoris, which also varies from woman to woman.

(7) The position of the clitoris may affect a woman's ability to reach orgasm through intercourse alone. The farther away from the mouth of the vagina the clitoris is, the less stimulation it receives during intercourse.

(8) During the height of arousal, the clitoris retreats demurely beneath its veil of skin rather than rearing up for all the world to see. It may even seem to disappear altogether, making it hard to find.

(9) A study on vaginal sensitivity found that the clitoris is nearly twice as sensitive to mild electric stimulation as the vaginal wall.

WHAT YOU NEED TO KNOW ABOUT HIS ORGASM

Life expectancy

Men who have orgasms twice a week double their chances of increasing their life expectancy.

Faking it

He can fake it. That's because ejaculation and orgasm are not the same thing.

Ejaculation

It is possible for men to have orgasms without ejaculating (think Tantric sex). Ejaculation is caused by a build up of sexual tension that causes the muscles near the prostate gland to contract. This sends the fluids from the prostate gland and seminal vesicles into the urethra, producing an 'Omigod, I'm coming' sensation (otherwise known as ejaculatory inevitability, or the neurological point of no return). In other words, he cannot suck those fluids back up into his glands and vesicles. While all this is going on, the brain is sending signals to close off the valve between the bladder and urethra and shoot the ejaculate down the urethra and out the penis. So this would more properly be described as the 'Omigod, I'm ejaculating' sensation – but that phrase is not as romantic to shout out.

Sexual tension

Orgasm is controlled by a different group of nerves in the spine. Like ejaculation, it is caused by a build-up of sexual tension. It is characterised by involuntary, rhythmic contraction of the pelvic muscles and usually some weird faces and grunting noises. This usually occurs around the time of ejaculation. But it can happen before or after.

Sexual peak

A man's desire for sex peaks in his late teens or early 20s. At this age he can have sex several times a day and his orgasms are explosive, intense and can last up to 30 seconds.

Forgetfulness

There's a medical reason he forgets your name – if he's over 70 years old. Strenuous sex can trigger 'transient global amnesia' or the Who the Hell Is This In Bed With Me? phenomenon. A good orgasm can create pressure in the brain's blood vessels, causing 12 to 24 hours of memory loss.

Post-sex coma

There's also a medical reason for his post-sex coma – and this one's for men of all ages. (It takes women 20 to 30 minutes to fall asleep after an orgasm, compared to the two to five before men pass out.) Oxytocin, a hormone responsible for the release of breast milk and supposedly for women's orgasmic contractions, also stimulates erection and ejaculation in men. Oxytocin is thought to cause drowsiness. But because women's bodies normally contain more of it, they may be less sensitive to its surges. Men get drunk on it. So even though both partners could feel the need to nod off due to their orgasm's release of tension and to bedtime fatigue, the wallop of an oxytocin cocktail is likely to make a man fall asleep first.

...And 3 Medical Orgasm Plugs

While the reason some women don't climax is most often psychological – such as not feeling comfortable with their partner or with sex in general – the problem is sometimes something your GP can help you with:

(1) There's no such thing as faulty equipment (not yours, anyway). Your vagina is not too big or too small for orgasm. Most women don't climax because they aren't getting the right kind and/or amount of stimulation. For some women it can take up to an hour, but who knows a man that lasts that long? Result: The woman doesn't have a chance to 'get hers'.

(2) Check your medicine cabinet. Antidepressants, anti-anxiety drugs and beta-blockers (prescribed for high blood pressure) can all prevent a woman from climaxing. Decongestants that dry out your sinuses can also dry the natural lubricant in your vagina. Your doctor can usually prescribe another drug or adjust your dosage.

(3) Get blooded. Arousal for women works the same way erection does for men: blood needs to flow to the pelvis. Blockages can be caused by any disease that causes vascular problems, such as diabetes, hypertension or heart disease. Try to lower your blood pressure through exercise and healthier food choices.

6 Non-Medical Things That Can Come Between You And Bliss

(1) You hate your body.

(2) You don't trust him as far as you can spit.

(3) You're mad as hell and you're not going to do it.

(4) Your faith or family are sitting on the edge of the bed, telling you shouldn't be doing this.

(5) You're too stressed to even think about sex.

(6) You're freaked because you're not having safe sex.

4 Ways to Permanently Deflate

(1) Doing pelvic floor exercises will strengthen vaginal muscles which in turn will help push the air out quicker (see Chapter Nine).

(2) Using lubrication will make things slick (see Chapter Six). The extra friction can cause excess air to build up, especially during rowdy sex.

(3) Slightly adjusting the angle at which the penis enters, by leaning a little farther backward or forward, can help.

(4) Certain positions, such as him-on-top and rear entry, seem to lend themselves to prime varting. Try having sex in a position that has a tighter seal and lets in less air. The woman on top position seems to reduce air build-up, while rear entry seems to enhance it.

Training Tips For Orgasming During Intercourse

(1) Use a vibrator or stimulate your clitoris during penetration.

(2) Use The Bridge: in this technique, your clitoris is touched up until the point of orgasm. His thrusting acts as the final trigger.

(3) Go Minimum Entry: your man gets on top and raising himself on his hands, ever so slightly moves his penis so that the tip is just barely moving in and out of your vagina. The rocking motion will create very pleasurable sensations. He then pushes all the way in just when you're on the brink of orgasm. Although this will be very arousing for you, it may not do as much for your partner as he would probably like.

(4) Maximum Withdrawal Technique works on the same principle, although it gives you a little less stimulation and your man a little more. In this, he pushes all the way in and then withdraws to the max. This will give both of you a full range of sensations with every stroke.

THE CARE AND FEEDING OF YOUR ORGASM

During sex my vagina sometimes makes an embarrassing noise. What is this?

It's nothing more than a little air on the loose. And it's called 'varts' (though perhaps not medically). Varting is what happens is during arousal, the vagina expands and the uterus moves, creating little air pockets. As you pass through excitement, the walls begin to collapse back to their normal state. Any air that got trapped in there will rush right back out in an unfortunate imitation of a whoopee cushion. Air can also be held and exhaled during penetrative or oral sex, depending on such things as your angle or on how you fit together with your partner.

> Women who do reach orgasm though intercourse alone may have a larger clitoris or one positioned so it is easily rubbed by a thrusting penis.

I find it very difficult to have an orgasm. I only seem to come if I'm on top. Nothing else works.

The inability to orgasm – or anorgasmia – is broken down into three categories:
Primary: you've never ever had the pleasure.
Secondary: you were a happy climaxer until one day the orgasms dried up.
Situational: you can only bliss out one way.

Unfortunately, the reasons for anorgasmia remain a big mystery. One thought is that women who suffer from it have been conditioned to think sex, in all its delicious forms, is bad or dirty.

Body image is another factor. If you don't think you're sexy, you're not going to feel sexual or be comfortable about having your body seen or touched. Other causes can include an unpleasant experience such as rape (see Chapter Six), painful intercourse, which may be due to vaginal infection, inadequate love play or pleasuring or related to a deteriorating relationship (see Pleasure Killers on p.106).

Or it could be a case of bad foreplay. Perhaps your partner is not hitting the right spot or getting the correct rhythm. This leads to anxiety which can deaden the feeling faster than your mother calling in the middle of sex.

More rarely, your lack of joy could be due to something physical (see 3 Medical Orgasm Plugs on p.101). The only way to get to the root of your problem is a doctor's visit to eliminate the above until you find out your personal orgasm decoder.

> You heartbeat revs to about 180 beats per minute during orgasm.

ORGASMS ARE NOT JUST FOR FUN

There may be a biological purpose to your pleasure:

- Scientists found that women who orgasm one minute before to 45 minutes after their lover ejaculates retain 80 per cent of his sperm, whereas very little sperm is stockpiled by women who orgasm outside that time limit or not at all.
- The rhythmic contractions after orgasm act as a big wave on which the sperm can surf up to the egg, encouraging fertilisation.
- If a woman feels pleasure from a lover, she is more likely to do it again, thus upping her chances of pregnancy with that person (if she isn't using contraception).

Sometimes my orgasms are very powerful and sometimes they are just okay. Why does that happen?

Orgasms are not like Big Macs: You can't be sure of getting the same product every time. Some orgasms may feel like no more than a pleasant flutter and others are of the peel-off-the-ceiling variety.

Certain physiological and psychological factors can muffle or perk up orgasm: your psychological or mental mood, your hormonal ebb and low, the amount and intensity of foreplay you've had, how many orgasms you've already had, and even the depth of penetration during intercourse.

Penis-in-vagina sex doesn't do it for me. What's wrong with me?

Welcome to the real world of sex. Only around 33 per cent of women are able to climax without additional stimulation. In fact, most women feel very little through the walls of the vagina most of the time, because the nerve cells located along the vaginal walls are not often activated or all that plentiful. (And the clitoris, the nerve centre of female pleasure, is located outside the vagina.)

This means what may be most pleasurable for men – the deep thrusting in and out motions of intercourse – may provide little sexual satisfaction for a woman. This doesn't mean you should just tolerate a visit from his penis. There are a few things you can try to maximise your pleasure:

Woman-on-top positions mean you can direct the pelvic thrusts towards stimulating your clitoris. Have him ride high: after he enters you, he moves upward and rests his pubic bone firmly against yours. As he thrusts, he'll rub your labia and, in turn, your clitoris. In one study, women who weren't regularly orgasmic reported an approximately 60 per cent increase in intercourse orgasms when they tried this trick.

Rear entry moves: this will let him use his hand or a vibrator on your clitoris while penetrating you.

WOMEN CAN GET PINK BALLS

Every time a person becomes sexually and genitally aroused, the penis or vulva fills with blood (vasocongestion). This is what makes his soldier stand to attention and gets your vagina pulsating in anticipation of a visitor. The orgasm and/or ejaculation for him means bye-bye vasocongestion – the swelling subsides and goes away.

But if you do not orgasm or ejaculate after sexual stimulation and arousal, vasocongestion sometimes sticks around like an unwanted house guest. The problem is that all that congested blood flow now has to reverse itself. Think of trying to empty a gallon of milk into a glass via a drinking straw – that's pretty similar to what is going on in your body.

In men, the pain is mainly felt in the testes (i.e. blue balls). Not because of a build-up of sperm (sperm doesn't build up that way), but because that's where many of the genital sensory nerves are. Women, on the other hand, may feel pain in the vulva or general pelvic area. The arousal will eventually fade away on its own. But to make the pain and swelling go away quickly, you want to get blood flowing. Here's how:

- The easiest way is to orgasm – either with a partner or through masturbation.
- Use a cold or warm compress or shower in cold water.
- Take an analgesic like ibuprofen or aspirin to alleviate the pain.
- Simple physical activity like running, walking or other sports will pump up circulation.
- Elevate the pelvis with a pillow for a spell to help drain the blood from the area and relieve pressure.

Is Your Contraception Getting In The Way Of Your Orgasm Or Helping It?

BIRTH CONTROL	BIG OH FACTOR!	MAKE IT HAPPEN
Diaphragm	1. The elastic ring can bash your cervix, causing pain. 2. The spermicide can cause allergic reaction. 3. May hinder access to the G-spot.	1. Make sure it fits properly. 2. Switch to Condoms. 3. Switch to the cervical cap.
Condoms	The latex or spermicide (if it's lubricated) can cause allergic reaction.	Switch brands
The Pill	The hormonal suppression can lower testosterone, causing a dip in desire.	Try a different hormonal mix.
Female Condom	Some women find that the ridge at the base of the female condom stimulates the clitoris during intercourse.	Enjoy!
Depo-Provera	Since this method significantly lowers oestrogen, lubrication may dwindle, affecting sexual pleasure. Testosterone drops and may suppress libido.	Try a different hormonal contraceptive.

Why do I always have to pee after sex?

The probing motion of the penis, a vibrator or a long finger can rub the bladder nerve endings on the vaginal wall. Once stimulated, these endings can make your bladder feel like it's about to let loose.

Some men also experience this feeling when similar sources apply pressure to the prostate (just inside the rectum). For both guys and gals, full bladders and bowels prior to playtime can intensify the urge to go during sex. So, urinating or excreting before engaging your sex tools can help reduce the sensation, or the actual need, to use the bathroom. Changing your sexual positions in order to find one where there is less pressure against your bladder, rectum, or prostate may also make a difference.

> For some women, sex brings on menstrual-like cramps. Such pain is a side effect of uterine contractions during intense orgasm and it generally lasts a short time (they can be headed off altogether with anti-inflammatory medication taken before sex starts).

After sex, I notice that my labia are quite swollen, to the point where my skin feels really tight. There is no pain but it worries me.

The extra blood flow to the pelvic area makes the labia engorged, just like the penis. The swelling can take a couple of hours to go away.

PLEASURE KILLERS

I often experience pain after orgasm. It can take about 15 minutes for my whole pelvic area to stop aching.

You could just be experiencing spasm of the muscles of the pelvic floor. This happens after a particularly intense orgasm. There's no cure other than skipping the orgasm altogether – and is the pain really that bad? A heating pad on your lower abdomen may help the pain go more quickly.

After I had sex, my vagina was bleeding and it stopped a few hours later. I didn't have my period.

Bleeding from the vaginal area following sexual intercourse is called post-coital bleeding. The amount of blood, how long it lasts and the number of times it happens may indicate how serious the problem is.

If it only happens once it is unlikely to be anything more than a slight tear in the vagina, caused during intercourse. This may produce just a small amount of discharge with blood in it.

However, persistent and heavy bleeding after intercourse needs to be checked out as it may be cancer (see Chapters Two and Three).

Sometimes I pee when I climax. Help!

Your bladder sits right above the vaginal area, so it can get stimulated during sex. Releasing urine during orgasm is common, as are foot spasms, involuntary pelvic thrusts and passing gas – see, it could be worse! It's all a natural part of letting go. Orgasm is, after all, a form of release. Try emptying your bladder before sex and doing pelvic floor exercises (see Chapter Nine) which strengthen the pelvic floor muscles and are used to treat urinary incontinence.

> In men the valve between the urethra and bladder shuts off during sex. This may cause some men to feel an urgent need to urinate.

Recently I've been experiencing excruciating pain in my head as I climax, leaving me almost in tears.

What you're having is a sex headache. Sex generally cures headaches, which makes it a poor excuse for skipping nookie. But for an unlucky few, sex with orgasm can cause two kinds of headaches. For some they are short in duration (five to ten minutes), while for others the pain can hang around for over an hour.

5 Questions That Can Be Answered In One Word

(1) **Does clitoral size make a difference to sensitivity?**

No

(2) **How many drinks on average will decrease orgasms?**

Two

(3) **What percentage of women have an orgasm during intercourse?**

30

(4) **What's the most likely way for a woman to reach orgasm?**

Masturbation

(5) **How many minutes should be spent on foreplay to make sure orgasm happens?**

21

this kind of headache could help minimise the pain. Taking a migraine medication that constricts blood vessels could also be helpful before you have sex.

Since I've been on the Pill, I haven't been able to have an orgasm, nor am I aroused during sex. What's going on?

You might want to try a different type of pill. Some types of birth control pills have a mini cold-water effect on your libido because their chemical make-up has a drying effect on lubrication. They also may decrease production of some pleasure-associated hormones (like androgen). Research suggests that the monophasic pill (which releases the same amount of hormones for 21 days – see Chapter Seven for more information) can decrease desire while the triphasic pill (which releases varying amounts of oestrogen and progestin over the month) has much less of an effect.

When I started taking antihistamines for allergies my orgasms disappeared. Could the two be related?

Absolutely. Some antihistamines can bungle sex in several ways. They dry up the mucus membranes that make allergies insufferable, putting an end to runny noses and all the paper hankies that go with them. But they can also dry up the vaginal lubrication that goes hand-in-hand with a woman's sexual arousal. They also have a sedating effect, which is supposed to knock you out and help you sleep after long nights of sniffling and sneezing. Finally, their numbing effect can make foreplay as frustrating as a fully fledged allergy attack.

In addition to these problems, anticholinergic antihistamines can trigger other unsettling side effects: confusion, light-headedness, dry mouth, constipation, and difficulty urinating. To sidestep these problems, switch to a non-sedating medication which will still quash your allergies but put your sex life back on track at the same time.

Most likely yours is a Coital cephalalgia, which develops when the blood vessels of the brain dilate and the muscles of the head and neck contract as orgasm approaches and your body tenses up. This headache is usually benign and rarely associated with a serious health problem. Taking a non-steroidal anti-inflammatory drug should give you some quick pain relief.

The second type of headache, known as Orgasmic cephalalgia or orgasmic headache, affects more men than women and is often experienced by people who have migraines. Typically felt around or behind the eyes, the pain often persists for a few minutes, but can continue up to several hours. Staying still while having

BOOKS

EXPANDED ORGASM: SOAR TO ECSTASY AT YOUR LOVER'S EVERY TOUCH
(Sourcebooks Inc, 2002)
by Patricia Taylor
A concise, how-to book on giving and receiving expanded orgasms. You and your partner are led through a step-by-step program, giving practical instructions that will help couples to connect in order to create an ecstatic new level of intimacy.

FIVE MINUTES TO ORGASM EVERY TIME YOU MAKE LOVE
(JPS Publications, 1998)
by Claire Hutchins
This is for any woman suffering the agonising frustration of an unreliable or non-existent orgasm. The text describes a method for making female orgasm the effortless outcome of each and every lovemaking experience.

THE BIG O: ORGASMS: HOW TO HAVE THEM, GIVE THEM, AND KEEP THEM COMING
(Broadway, 2001)
by Lou Paget
The most essential and cutting-edge information explaining – with step-by-step instructions – all you want to know about orgasms.

HOW TO GIVE HER ABSOLUTE PLEASURE: TOTALLY EXPLICIT TECHNIQUES EVERY WOMAN WANTS HER MAN TO KNOW
(Broadway, 2000)
by Lou Paget
Based on the secrets shared by hundreds of men and women in Paget's enormously popular seminars, this book gives the true scoop on what women really like, and why, along with detailed surefire techniques. Complete with step-by-step illustrations, as well as a catalogue of sex toys and tips on how to use them.

TANTRIC ORGASM FOR WOMEN
(Inner Traditions International, 2004)
by Diana Richardson
A revolutionary approach to female sexuality that focuses on relaxation as the key to achieving deep orgasmic states.

FEMALE MASTURBATION : EVERY WOMAN'S ORGASM IS UNIQUE
(Director: The Welcomed Consensus)
This DVD is highly informational for both men and women as it shows a simple, uncut film of a woman from a low state of arousal to a heightened, extended orgasm with many close-up shots of her genitalia. The viewer can witness all of the signs of orgasm in her body, as well as the details of her technique that anyone can use to better their sex lives with their partner.

SEX TIPS FOR GIRLS
(Channel 4 Books, 2002)
by Flic Everett
This book has loads of ideas.

THE BLUFFER'S GUIDE TO SEX: BLUFF YOUR WAY IN SEX
(Oval Books, 1999)
by Sarah Brewer and Tim Webb
A short, basic book that covers a lot of ground, by a UK doctor.

INFORMATION AND ADVICE

For Dr Grafenberg's Original article on the G-Spot, log onto
http://doctorg.com/Grafenberg.htm
You've read about it, poked around for it –
now you can go to the original source.

www.urologychannel.com/fsd/index.shtml
For information on various causes of female
sexual dysfunction including diagnosis and
treatment, go to the website.

www.femalefirst.co.uk/relationships/
Female Firsts relationships channel has a
good range of features about women and sex,
and some down-to-earth Q&As to give you even
more ideas.

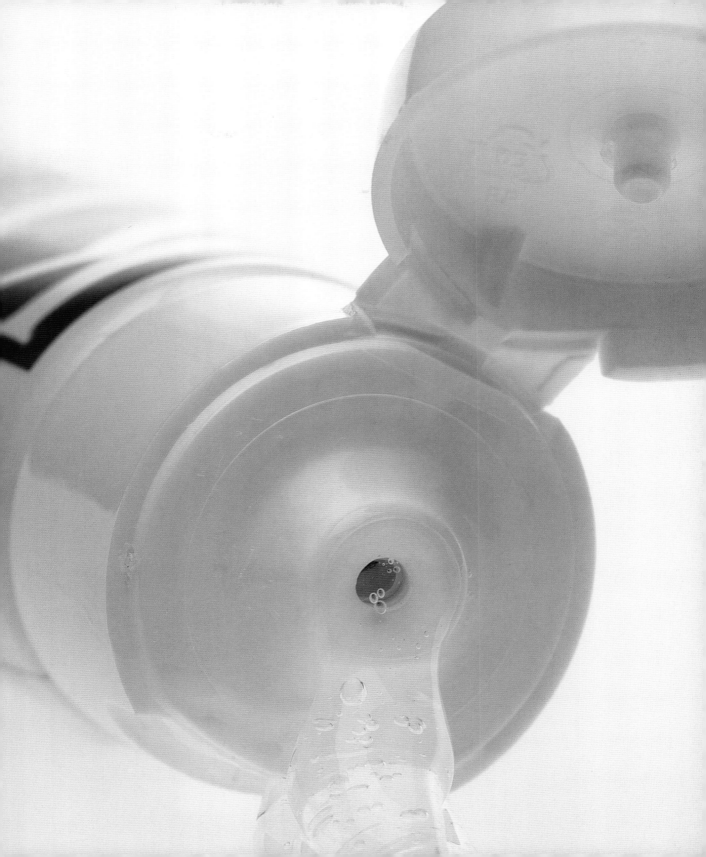

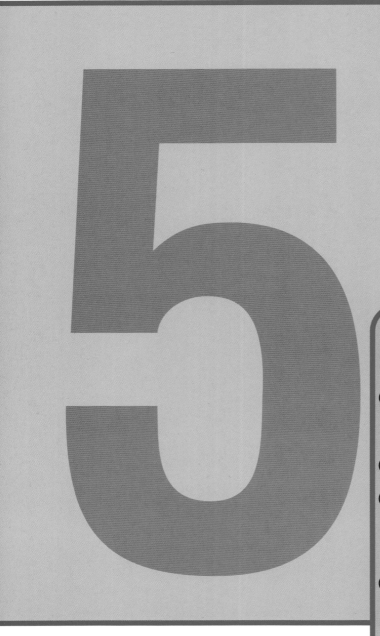

5 Libido Health habits

(1) A Viagra pill is consumed every three seconds somewhere in the world. Yet if men exercised for about 20 minutes a day, they'd lower their chances of ever becoming impotent.

(2) Use it or lose it: sex acts as desire insurance (yes, masturbation counts).

(3) If you're planning on a romantic dinner, have sex before, not as afters. Although most people think a big meal will put you in the mood, digesting actually drains energy, especially if you add wine, since alcohol is a depressant.

(4) Beware of the hormonal supplement melatonin, sold as a sleep aid. It's been rumoured to enhance sex drive but actually does the opposite.

(5) Avoid caffeine within eight hours of bedtime – it inhibits sleep (which in turn inhibits desire) and also acts as a downer on the libido.

EQUIPMENT FAILURE

Everything you need to know when things go wrong.

When your sexual parts are not functioning as you would like them to 'Ouch!' is not, for most people, a huge turn-on. The same goes for 'y-a-w-n' or 'Oops!' When the process of sex breaks down, it can turn the whole thing into one big sorry-I've-got-a-headache. But before you blame the relationship (or the size of your thighs), check you health. Then check his. Some fairly mundane – and easily correctable – medical conditions can make sex unsatisfying, unworkable or simply uninteresting. This chapter gives the common sexual saboteurs, how to spot them, when to worry and what to do so that matters don't go from bad to worse.

MOOD BUSTERS

Since my boyfriend put on weight he doesn't seem as good.

His extra weight may be getting in the way – literally. The fat pad just above the penis can become enlarged and cover up the penis somewhat. So while his penis isn't any shorter, there's probably less penetration.

He doesn't like using spermicide

The mix can be lethal: the skin on the penis and scrotum is one of the most absorptive skin surfaces on the body and the active ingredient of spermicides is necessarily highly toxic in order to kill the sperm. Try different brands, as he may be more sensitive to the inactive ingredients in one cream or jelly than another.

Minimising contact with spermicide should help too. Trying a non-spermicide condom alone or a diaphragm where most of the spermicide is inside the device might also ease his discomfort.

DO YOU NEED A SHRINK?

Firstly, some clarification: you do not have sex in sex therapy. That is sex surrogacy and much less common. Psychosexual Therapy helps with most sexual problems that haven't been resolved with time or medication. The troubles fit into three basic categories: can't get it up, can't get it in, can't be bothered.

You can go on your own or with your partner. To begin with, you talk with the therapist to try to work out if the root of your problem is physical, psychological or a mix of the two. Then your therapist will give you homework, usually a customised plan of exercises for you (and your partner if you've got one) to do at home. The point of these exercises is to help you feel more comfortable sexually.

Do women have testosterone like men?

Yes, although there are two differences in how testosterone works with women:

● Women have less of it.
● It is produced by the adrenal glands and the ovaries, with the ovaries probably the most important source.

However, testosterone definitely has an effect on the female gotta-have-it response. Besides causing your nipples and clitoris to become erect, a recent study of sexually active women showed a significant correlation between blood testosterone levels and sexual responsiveness and satisfaction.

I have completely gone off sex. I don't even fantasise.

Sexual appetite tends to wax and wane. There are periods in your life when you have little desire for sex, and other periods when sex assumes an overriding importance. Most of the time you are somewhere in between. So losing interest in sex is probably a temporary phase and not a disaster.

It's normal to lose interest in sex temporarily when things are crazy at work/if you're bereaved/you've got the flu/you've got a cold sore/your hormones are out of kilter, plus the one hundred million other things that can stress you or your body out and make sex the last thing on your mind.

This isn't the end of the road. These sexual dry spells are merely a roadblock. Once work has calmed down/you've mourned your loss/you're feeling well again/you found out the cold sore wasn't herpes/your hormones are more balanced, and so on, you will usually regain an interest in sex after a couple of months.

But when it's been months or you find yourself thinking you wouldn't be bothered if you never had sex again – there may be a problem that needs further medical investigation (see Sex Headaches on p.118).

WHAT'S YOUR
PROBLEM?

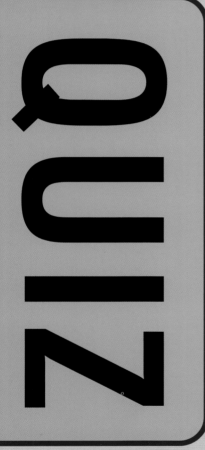

QUESTIONS

① **Sexual dysfunction is generally what kind of problem?**
a Physical
b Emotional
c Psychological

② **Viagra works for women True or False?**

③ **Which of the following doesn't affect arousal?**
a Heart disease
b Prescription drugs
c Depression
d Smoking
e Antibiotics

④ **Which of the above is most likely to cause sexual problems?**

⑤ **Which of the following three groups runs the lowest risk for sexual problems?**
a Younger women
b Older men

ANSWERS

1 (a) Research in the last three to five years shows that impotence or sexual dysfunction is largely a physical problem. Sexual dysfunction could be a sign of cardiovascular conditions, depression, anxiety or prostate problems. It could also be an early warning sign of a heart attack.

2 False. The sex mechanisms are different for women and initial studies have found that Viagra does not have an effect on women.

3 (e) While antibiotics may have a connection with thrush, which can act like a dehydrator on lubrication, they don't actually have an effect on desire.

4 (b) Prescription medications are a leading cause of sexual dysfunction.

5 (b) Older men, followed by younger women with older women bringing up the rear. For older men (and women), the problems are primarily physical; for younger women, the problems are primarily psychological.

Not Tonight, honey...

Here are proven solutions from three different approaches to five common arousal problems. The point is, desire is a mysterious thing. And often there are all sorts of reasons for not being in the mood.

PROBLEM	PRESCRIPTION		
	MEDICAL	NATURAL	SEX THERAPIST
Too tired.	See your GP.	Take ginseng (see Chapter Seven).	Set aside some prime time for sex.
'I have a headache.'	Take two ibuprofen.	Have sex. It's been found to cure aches and pains.	Skip it.
PMS	Take two ibuprofin.	Drink tea made from dong quai root.	Have an orgasm – it helps alleviate PMS (see Chapter Four).
'I'm stressed out.'	Do aerobics.	Do Tantric sex.	Sex is an excellent stress reliever.
'I'm not good in bed.'	See a psychotherapist.	Take Chinese polygala root for sexual confidence.	Think erotic, not neurotic.

My boyfriend never wants to have sex anymore.

There are many things that can put the crimp in a guy's sex drive within a relationship, including everything from depression, to guilt over some action (such as he slept with his boss), to low hormone levels, to substance abuse, to getting his needs met somewhere else (again, such as he slept with his boss), to he's not crazy about you, to he's unsure about the relationship, to working too hard… you get the picture. BTW, these things can cool you too (see Sex Headaches on p.118).

Acupuncture has been found to help push sex drive.

The only way to know for sure is to start talking and decide if you need to:

● Help him de-stress.
● Make an appointment with his GP.
● Hold off on ordering bridal magazines.
● Break up with him.

LUBE JOB

What is lubrication?

It's intercourse sauce. Wetness is the orgasm's secret ingredient; without it, your love experience will have the same pleasure factor as a trip to the dentist without Novocaine.

When a woman becomes aroused, she starts experiencing vasocongestion, which is basically the same process that makes his penis stand up and take notice. Vasocongestion causes the clitoris and breasts to swell and the vaginal cavity to expand, and it also signals for those love juices to start flowing. In this 'sweating' process, called transudation, clear fluid or plasma seeps though the membrane of the vaginal walls as the engorging blood vessels that lie between its cells squeeze the liquid out. The combination of vaginal mucus and lubrication makes up women's sexual secretions, which can contain carbohydrates, amino acids, proteins, and other acids produced by the normal lactobacillus bacteria.

I often feel dry during sex, even though I'm horny. I'm nowhere near the menopause, so what's wrong?

A woman's vagina simply does not produce an unlimited flow of lubricant like some sexual tap, even if she is being turned on. When it's a desert down there, a few things might be the culprit and you may have to experiment to find the solution.

What's the best lubrication to use?

Here's a primer for picking out a motion lotion.

● Stay away from oils as vagina greasers. Petroleum jelly is likely to remain coating the vaginal walls for days, welcoming all kinds of bacteria and creating an environment that promotes thrush (see Chapter Two). In fact, all oils will linger in your vagina and entire genital region longer than you wish, as there is no way for them to be flushed out of your body. And oils of any kind will destroy latex condoms, gloves, caps and diaphragms faster than you can say, 'Hole-y smoke!', making them less effective in protecting against pregnancy and STDs.

One study of happily married couples found that when it came to sex, 50% of the men reported a lack of interest or an inability to relax.

● Stick with silicone. It's thin, sticky, and slippery – in other words, most like your own natural wetness.
● Skip the extra flavour. Water-based lubricants are especially formulated to be taste-free, non-staining, non-irritating to genital tissue and they will easily wash out of your body. They contain de-ionized (purified) water, long chain polymers (biologically inert plastics commonly found in foods and cosmetics) and some kind of preservative ingredient to prevent contamination by viruses and bacteria. Remember, the more added ingredients in a lubricant,

SEX HEADACHES

Here are 22 surprising sex saboteurs you do, use, abuse, or encounter in daily life.

The drug factor

- Marijuana in small occasional doses can heighten the senses and make sex more pleasurable, but overuse might similarly destroy sex drive.
- Antidepressants can make testosterone levels take a dive by raising serotonin levels.
- Diet drugs often contain mood-altering ingredients (such as caffeine) that keep you from relaxing and other ingredients that interfere with the arousal process.
- Sedatives and sleep aids can also put your sex life to sleep. Any drug that causes you to become drowsy or warns you against operating heavy machinery isn't going to help you do any heavy lifting in bed.
- Some prescription drugs, such as Beta blockers for cardiovascular disease, ulcer and heartburn H2 blockers, cholesterol medications, high blood pressure medication and pills to prevent migraines, can cause decreased libido in both sexes and impotence in men.
- Even the most seemingly innocent medicines, such as certain prescription eye drops, acne medicines, antacids, antihistamines and anti-inflammatories, can inhibit desire by interfering with the body's chemistry.

The solution: usually within each class of drugs is an alternative that may have minimal or no side effects on sex drive. If you think the drug you are taking is interfering with your sex life, ask your doctor about switching. If you're taking an antidepressant, ask your doctor about weekend 'drug holidays', where patients take a temporary break from the medication (say, from Thursday morning through Sunday night).

The disease factor

- Clinical depression affects your libido as well as your psyche. Surveys show that about two out of three people with depression lose interest in sex, as a result of imbalances in brain biochemistry.

The solution: therapy and/or subscribed antidepressants. But beware, the cure can be worse that the disease – see the The Drug Factor, left.

The hormone factor

- Anything that can put your hormones out of kilter can wreak havoc on your sex life: menstruation, oral contraceptives, pregnancy, childbirth, the menopause, crash diets, excessive exercise, chemotherapy or a hysterectomy may all cause a drop in oestrogen. This can lead to a lack of vaginal lubrication and a loss of sex drive. Some women experience a drop in testosterone.

The solution: depending on which way the hormonal pendulum is swinging, your doctor may prescribe hormone replacement therapy or tell you to look at your diet.

The mental factor

- Everyday stress has been shown to take a toll on sexual desire. Stress can hinder sex drive, because stress reduces testosterone levels in both sexes. Moreover, the stress hormone adrenalin shunts blood flow away from the genitals.

- An unpleasant past experience can affect the present; this can include memories of sexual abuse or a relationship that went wrong.
- Worrying, especially about sexual matters (such as contraception, STDs, sexual abilities) can trigger a loss of interest in sex.
- Your self-esteem is on holiday. If you're not feeling good about yourself then you're going to find it difficult to see yourself as a sexual person.
- It's not you – it's him. If you're feeling angry, upset or in any way insecure about your relationship, then you need to deal with these issues before you can expect to feel like getting naked with him.

The solution: sex therapy (see Do You Need A Shrink? on p.114)

The life factor
- Too little sleep can cause too little sex drive. Scientists have yet to tease apart the sex-sleep connection, but it's likely that the hormone vasopressin, which helps regulate body temperature, plays a role.
- Too much exercise can backlash in the bedroom. While about an hour a day will give you a hormonal zing (and being in shape can make you feel terrific), more than that on a regular basis can mess with monthly hormonal cycles in women and men.
- Too much dieting puts desire on a diet. Research shows that a brain chemical called neuropeptide Y, which kicks into high gear in response to food deprivation, also undermines sex drive.
- Conversely, fatty foods can cause testosterone levels to drop.

- A new baby. Think about it: it demands time and energy; meanwhile hormone balances are changing and there may be soreness from stitches. Around 50 per cent of women do not have much interest in sex for around three months after childbirth.
- Using highly scented soaps and perfumes can interfere with your ability to detect male scent, which can have a cold water effect on your libido.
- Going off your lover can turn you off.
- Perhaps they're not a very skilled lover and the whole experience simply does nothing for you. Or they're doing or saying something in bed that makes you feel uncomfortable.

The solution: lead a healthy lifestyle – eat healthily and exercise in moderation, avoid caffeine and too much booze, get at least seven hours of shut-eye a night, wait out some of the temporary stresses and only go to bed with someone you're attracted to. If none of these work, sexual therapy may be in order.

The contraception factor
- Some contraceptives that contain progestogen (Depo-Provera) can depress your natural sex drive. The birth control may be working, but not in the way intended.
- Monophasic pills, which keep the body in a static hormonal state, can act as a downer on sex drive.

The solution: change your contraception. For instance, triphasic pills, which deliver steadily increasing doses of hormones across the cycle, have been found to boost desire.

The Lube Factor

THE DEHYDRATOR	HOW TO MOISTURISE
You're not sufficiently aroused.	Spend at least 30 minutes on foreplay.
Lubrication is normally lowest a day or two before your period.	Use extra lubrication for a couple of days before your period.
Illnesses resulting in dryness.	Thyroid disease (see Chapter Three), thrush (see Chapter Two) and Bacterial Vaginosis (see Chapter Two).
nonoxynol-9 spermicide in condoms can cause irritation and even burning which can result in dryness.	Switch to a non-lubricated condom.
The Pill and Depo-Provera (by changing your hormonal levels), antidepressants (by affecting your libido), and antihistamines and decongestants (by drying up mucous), acne treatments (they contain dehydrating agents).	Check your medicine cabinet and see if you can switch brands.
Using alcohol, any amphetamine and/or marijuana before and during sex can dehydrate vaginal secretions.	Treat your body like a temple.
Pregnancy and breastfeeding cause hormonal fluctuations.	Use extra lubrication.
Stress can throw almost any natural physical response off kilter.	Try relaxation techniques and stock up on extra lubrication.

the greater your chances of having an allergic reaction or developing an infection (and the genital area is not one that you want to expose to rashes).

- Skip the spermicide. Some lubes contain the sperm assassin nonoxynol-9, which can irritate the vagina, making sex uncomfortable. These also have a somewhat soapy flavour and may even briefly numb your tongue (see Chapter Eight for more nonoxynol-9 dangers).

I was having sex when this liquid came gushing out of me. It wasn't pee, but it made a huge wet spot.

Now you know what a guy feels like. Actually, female ejaculation is pretty similar to semen (without the sperm, of course), with high levels of prostatic acid phosphatase (as well as glucose). Like semen, it comes from the Skene's glands, prostate-like glands located in a woman's urethra. Most female ejaculators let fluid flow to the tune of about one teaspoon, though evidence of some female ejaculate can be found in almost any woman's love juices after sexual stimulation.

> Avoid the limited chemist lube selection and head for your friendly neighbourhood adult toy store. They have a wider variety, including flavoured and creamier versions.

PAIN KILLERS

I sometimes get a pain in my legs in the middle of sex, to the point where I have to jump up and hop around.

That can really put a cramp on your style. Sometimes lovemaking can feel as if you're having a tryst with a treadmill. You may experience nasty cramps in your legs and the pain can be so bad that you are forced to stop, stand up and massage your legs, which of course completely destroys your momentum.

No matter how toned you are, leg and foot muscles can get strained when you're in the missionary position. Dehydration, fatigue or even an overheated room can intensify the problem. Kneading the muscles is the only remedy, so have your partner lend a hand to keep the sex vibes going.

If your thighs tend to cramp mid-action, try this stretch beforehand: sitting on the floor, bring soles of feet together; gently press thighs down for a count of ten; relax and repeat.

To avoid calf aches, steady yourself against a wall with both hands; place your right foot in front of you with knee bent, and place your left leg about two feet behind you, keeping it straight. Press your left heel towards the floor. Repeat on the opposite side. To prevent foot cramps, sit with your legs straight ahead; point and flex your toes several times.

We were experimenting with a new postion when I hurt my back.

Any position that involves a lot of bending, usually the case for whoever's on top or for both partners during rear entry, places the back at risk for injury. If yours starts to hurt while making love, stop immediately. This is not a no pain, no gain situation. Place an ice pack on the area, then lie on your side with the knees bent and a pillow between them; an over-the-counter anti-inflammatory pain medication can also help.

To stop spasms and prevent stiffness, do some gentle stretches, such as resting on your back and hugging your knees to your chest. For the first 48 hours after an injury, apply an ice pack for 15 minutes, three times a day and have your partner work in a muscle rub – see, it's not all bad! After two days, use a heating pad for 15 minutes four times a day. If the pain persists after 48 hours, or if you experience numbness in your legs, get to the doctor as you may have a more serious internal injury.

> Around 58% of women regularly ejaculate about one teaspoon of fluid.

Whenever I have sex, that little area between my vagina and my bottom hurts.

That angry inch of yours is called the 'perineum'. The first thing you should do is take some time off from sexual intercourse. A cut down there is like a paper cut; it takes at least a few weeks to heal. When you do get back on your bronco, make sure you use plenty of lubrication to prevent further tears.

It feels like the penis is hitting something and hurting me on the inside when I have sex.

It sounds like you may have a tilted uterus. Think of your body as a motorway with constant roadworks – at the point where the cervical canal feeds into the uterus, there is an exit ramp called the cervico-uterine junction. Sometimes, for reasons unknown (which is pretty much the case with all roadworks), there is a slight detour in the system where the uterus bends a little. A uterus may tip forward towards the abdomen and the bladder (anteverted), which happens in about 80 per cent of uterus tilts. Or a uterus may tilt back towards the back and rectum (retroverted), which is also a normal variation, similar to being left-handed instead of right-handed.

About 30 per cent of women have some sort of displacement of their uterus, most without symptoms. Generally, it's no big deal – like having a bump in your nose. But for a few unlucky tipsters (like you), sex can be a bumpy ride because the penis pushes against the uterus, acting like a battering ram. This puts pressure on the rectum and ligaments of the tailbone.

Changing sexual position and/or the angle of his dangle when he penetrates you can ease your pain.

> Stress and lack of foreplay are thought to be two of the largest causes of vaginismus.

Sex has suddenly started to hurt. The muscles at the entrance to my vagina feel as if they are going into spasm, to the point where my partner can't penetrate me.

The vagina has a sphincter, a grouping of muscles that controls its tightness. This sphincter relaxes to allow things to get in (penises, fingers, doctor's speculums, and tampons) and out (babies). When the sphincter clenches and shuts down, preventing all forms of penetration, it's called vaginismus. Just as you'd clench your hands or jaw if someone tried to force something inside when you didn't want, so your vaginal muscles are protecting you by tensing.

Although rare, vaginismus can make sex either excruciatingly painful or impossible. And the reason it happens can be very different for each woman: it can result from some unresolved sexual conflict, such as sexual abuse or a belief that sexual activity is generally undesirable. You may have had a painful vaginal condition like endometriosis (see Chapter Two) that has left you with a conditioned fear of sex. You may be angry at your partner, causing you to close down when he tries to penetrate you.

> Some women with vaginismus can insert a tampon without any problem, but others find that trying to insert anything at all – a tampon, a finger, a penis – makes the muscles contract.

Most vaginismus is temporary and is relieved through self-help (see Pain, Pain, Go Away, opposite).

If you experience recurring or chronic vaginismus, you may need sexual therapy to find out what is causing your distress and to learn how to relax your vaginal muscles during sex.

Vaginal trainers may also help; these come as a set of four smooth penile-shaped cones, which are graduated in size and length. Working through the size grades helps relax your vagina in anticipation of penetration.

PAIN, PAIN, GO AWAY!

If you are in pain experiment with the following:
- Try de-stressing: Take deep breaths, relaxing your entire body on the out-breath. Do this ten times.
- Warm packs or relaxing baths might help relax you.
- Lots, lots and even more foreplay – the more the vagina is caressed, the more blood flow is brought to the area, adding to arousal, which leads to a general involuntary loosening of vaginal muscles in preparation for penetration.
- Have an orgasm from cunnilingus before intercourse to relax those muscles.

Is it normal to experience pain during intercourse?
- Sex should never be painful. If you are having pain during sex (dyspareunia), stop. A number of things could cause you to say, 'Ouch!':

If it hurts when he tries to penetrate it could be:
- Vaginitis (see Chapter Two).
- Your vagina is too dry (see Lube Factor on p.120).
- You have thrush (see Chapter Two) or herpes (see Chapter Eight), which is making the vulva sore.
- You have blocked Bartholin's glands (these help produce lubrication for sex), causing a cyst (see Chapter Two).
- Vulvodynia (see Chapter Two).

The pain is deep inside during sex, it could be:
- Pelvic Inflammatory Disease (PID, see Chapter Eight).
- Endometriosis (see Chapter Three).
- Pelvic Pain Syndrome: For two out of every three women with deep pain during sex, no cause can be found; you may have to accept that you have pelvic pain syndrome. This syndrome is not fully understood, but it is related to stress.
- Not enough foreplay (so you're not fully aroused).
- Small amounts of air could be getting trapped within the vaginal canal.
- The penis is hitting your cervix.
- You're sore from too much sex.
- You pulled your pelvic sling muscle.
- You have tears in the ligaments that support the uterus.
- He is unusually well endowed.

Bottom line: sex hurts and it shouldn't. See a doctor to find out why.

When my boyfriend penetrates me fully, it is very painful inside. Is there something wrong with me or is his penis too long?
He wishes. The vagina is extremely stretchy (after all, a baby has to fit through there at some point), but deep penetration can put tension on the ligaments and nerves at the far end. Keep sex slow and gentle when he's on top and try altering your position. Side entry – when you lie in front of him on your side – may be more comfortable because penetration won't be as deep.

If the pain persists, have your doctor check you out for a physical problem such as PID (see Chapter Eight), vaginismus, chronic constipation, bowel disorders or endometriosis (see Chapter Three) – all of which can affect how it feels when he crosses your threshold.

I recently had a pretty intense night of sex. My vagina has hurt ever since.
Marathon sex can leave a painful souvenir: vaginal tears or ulcerations. These cuts will usually heal on their own within a few days, but make sure you

HE HURTS TOO

Women aren't the only ones who experience pain. A few things can make a man cry out (and not in pleasure) during sex:

- Tight foreskin (see Chapter Four).
- Any lesion on the skin of the penis (due to unlubricated masturbation, rapid intercourse or STDs).
- Herpes blisters.
- Peyronie's disease.
- Penile fracture.

He likes rear position, but it hurts me. Is this normal?
Look at the mechanics: rear – or doggy-style – position lets him penetrate you as deeply as possible (which is why he likes it). But it's that deep penetration that causes the pain. Two possibilities: first, mix in some lubrication to help minimise friction (see Lube Factor on p.120); and secondly, have him inch his way in rather than deep plunging. This will let your body get used to the penetration.

practice ultra-safe sex during that time as the tears make you more vulnerable to STDs. In the meantime, soothe the pain with a warm bath, cold compresses and an over-the-counter ointment specifically made for vaginal use.

Whenever I have sex, it burns
There are a few possibilities:
- A reaction to a new brand of spermicide or latex condom.
- A vaginal infection: the most common is group B, strep vaginitis, which is easily treated with antibiotics.
- You're not lubricated enough during sex and that's

causing microscopic tears on your vaginal wall. These tears happen all the time, but the friction can cause burning in some people.
- You have an STD like chlamydia (see Chapter Eight).The only way to know for sure what's burning down your house is to get checked out by a doctor.

ERECTOR SETS

How long does it take for him to get hard again after ejaculation?
His recharging time – called the refractory period – varies from man to man. Basically, this is downtime for his penis after all the muscle contractions his system went through to bring semen and its sperm from the testes through the penis to its destination. For some men, it's mere minutes before they can come again; for others, it takes hours, or a good night's sleep. Generally, the younger he is, the sooner his penis will be ready to come out and play.

My boyfriend takes a long time to get hard. Is there a way to speed him up? (Everything works fine once he's erect.)
When you want to ignite him quickly, you need to get the blood flowing more quickly to his love zone. There are a few 'quickies' that should do the trick:
- Stimulating the prostate gland directly (see Chapter Six).
- Cupping his testicles and pressing them gently towards his body; this mimics the moves his body makes involuntarily right before orgasm.
- Squeeze his entire penis. This sends a message to his brain that blood is needed there – fast.

A man who is otherwise aroused but slow to rise may have a circulatory problem – he should get his blood sugar level checked for diabetes as well as a blood pressure and cholesterol test.

Lately, when my boyfriend and I have any sexual contact it's over before I can blink. This isn't normal for him. What's wrong?

Sounds like he has a bad case of PE (premature ejaculation). This is a very common problem (affecting up to 40 per cent of men) in which a man feels that he has no control over the timing of his orgasm and ejaculation.

It can happen at any time in his life. Rarely a cause for medical concern, premature ejaculation can suddenly appear due to over-excitement, age, stress, a lack of interest and/or fatigue – all moments when he has less control over his body.

However, if his PE is more or less a permanent feature of your lovemaking, it may be more chronic. The root causes go back to the way men learn to orgasm, which is typically through masturbation. A lot of young boys masturbate quickly, because they don't want someone to walk in on them. In other words, it's a learned behaviour – which means that it can become unlearned by gaining control of the pelvic muscles that govern orgasm. Habitual PE'ers never develop a normal sense of what their genitals feel like when they are highly excited and about to come. They need to learn how to tune into their bodies so that they begin to recognise the point of no return.

There are a number of techniques he can try to help him retrain and regain control. Most of these he can practice on his own as well:

- The Big Squeeze: when he thinks he's about to lose it, hold the shaft of his penis in your hand. Give it a firm squeeze for a count of ten. That should be enough to temporarily delay his urge to explode.
- Stop-Start: similar to above only instead of squeezing when he's on the brink, just stop stimulation until the feeling subsides (usually 30 seconds) and then resume. Repeat a few times.

> Studies show that while using anabolic steroids helps men have twice as many erections, they have trouble maintaining the erection during sex and climaxing.

- Breathing Bonus: taking deep breaths are the secret to Tantric sex and you know how long that can last. When he feels an orgasm approaching, he should stay very still with his penis still in penetration position. Then, relaxing his genital muscles, he takes a long breath in through his nose for a count of five seconds and holds it for two. Then he exhales through his mouth for six seconds. Once he feels in control, he can start moving again, slowly.

> If his penis has turned to stone even when he's not aroused, he may have priapism, a condition in which a male develops a permanent erection.

5 Questions That Can Be Answered In One Word

1. **How soon should a healthy man be able to repeat intercourse?**
   30 minutes

2. **Which is the most common sexual problem among men aged 18-59?**
   PE

3. **For a sexual difficulty to be considered a 'problem' or 'dysfunction', roughly how often should it be happening?**
   25 per cent of the time

4. **When is the best time to have sex?**
   Morning

5. **What causes arousal physically?**
   Blood

Mind Games

6 Non-medical things that can cause him to lie down and play dead:

(1) There might be something on his mind (poor penis performance in the past, job anxiety, your best friend), which will affect the penis' performance.

(2) There might be something on his mind that has caused his shrink to prescribe Seroxat, Zoloft, Prozac or any of a number of antidepressants which, while having a beneficial effect on his mood, can shut down the equipment for the duration of usage.

(3) He's really tired.

(4) He's really drunk.

(5) He's intimidated by you and your sex goddess qualities.

(6) Something you did had an adverse effect on him, such as calling him the wrong name, or something you didn't do, such as wash!.

- Suit Up: one more good reason to burn rubber; a condom can help reduce the sensation (as any man will tell you). Studies show that men who wear condoms during sex last about three minutes longer than guys who ride bareback.
- Take care of business first: masturbating first a couple of hours before making love can result in an increased ability to last longer.
- Change your position: changing positions every so often can also help, perhaps by giving the man brief pauses during lovemaking every now and then. Missionary seems to lend itself to moving fast; you on top seems to slow the action down. If he only wants to be on top, he can try pressing his pelvic bone against yours and rocking rather than thrusting his body. It won't be as stimulating for him, so he'll last longer, and it may be more stimulating for you.

- Go numb: desensitising creams contain a mild anaesthetic (7.5 per cent benzocaine) that causes a temporary numbing sensation after being applied to the skin. Although this lengthens staying power for many men, it comes with a price: most of these men said that the cream also makes sex less pleasurable. Unfortunately, the dulling effect can be transferred and felt by you, making it take longer for you to reach orgasm, not usually the desired effect.
- Give the pelvis a workout. Pelvic floor exercises aren't just for women (see Chapter Nine).
- Ball up: as he gets more and more aroused, his testicles move up toward his body. By pulling them back down, you can delay orgasm. Gently take hold of his scrotum just above the testicles. Then tug gently.
- Think about anything but sex, such as work, football scores, household chores – concentrating on anything non-sexual may hinder ejaculation.
- Change his diet: make his love last. Caffeine, alcohol and spicy foods can irritate the prostate and affect his staying power.

After a few drinks he can't get it up. Should he switch to low-alcohol lager?

When it comes to sex, it seems that a stiff drink can have quite the opposite effect on his body. Alcohol can dull the libido as well as his ability to obtain an erection. It acts on the central nervous system to depress the area of the brain where libido originates, as well as perhaps having an effect on penile blood flow itself.

If Erection Deficiency (ED) is more of a constant than a come-and-go visitor, he needs to be checked out for other serious medical problems. The condition has been found to be an early-warning signal of heart disease and stroke.

WILL HE GO LIMP ON YOU?

Is he under 30?
Arteries narrow and restrict blood flow with age.

Is he in good health?
Diabetes, high blood pressure and cholesterol are major erection busters, see Erection Killers His Doctor Can Cure on p.128. Being overweight increases his risk for these conditions.

Is he a low-stress person?
A brain overwhelmed by stress, anxiety, fatigue, or other mental concerns is less likely to send out the 'Let's party!' signal. Chronic high stress also elevates blood pressure, which constricts blood flow.

Does he eat like a pig?
Fibre helps keep vessels clear, weight healthy and lowers cholesterol, keeping him erect longer. Fatty foods have the opposite effect, contributing to arterial plaque and slowing down blood flow.

Does he get his bum off the sofa?
Exercise helps shed pounds, lower blood pressure and cholesterol, and keeps blood vessels healthy, including those critical ones in the groin area.

Are cotton buds the only thing in his medicine chest?
Common drugs such as antihistamines, appetite suppressants and blood pressure medications can affect the nerve impulses that lead to erection. The same goes for medication for depression, insomnia and kidney and liver diseases.

Is his liver pure?
Binge drinking can cause an ED episode that leads to performance anxiety.

Does he have clean lungs?
Smoking burns erections by constricting blood vessels throughout the body.

Is he calm?
Chronic feelings of anger and hostility spike blood pressure.

Is he a happy-go-lucky guy?
Studies find that depressed men are more likely to experience ED. And antidepressants also work against the libido, limiting his inclination to get erect in the first place.

Does he use it?
Research confirms that you've got to use it if you don't want to lose it. Having and using erections helps keep his penis in working order.

Is he a confident lover?
He doesn't have to be 007, but worry over past failure can cause future ones.

Does he stay out of the saddle?
Saddle sports like cycling, motorcycling, horseback riding can cause impact trauma, resulting in ED.

The more 'no' answers, the more at risk he is of ED.

ERECTION KILLERS HIS DOCTOR CAN (PROBABLY) CURE

Certain medical conditions may be putting a damper on his erection. The older he is, the more likely his ED is because of one of the following:

ERECTIONS KILLERS

Illnesses

- Diabetes, kidney disease, Peyronie's Disease, chronic alcoholism, multiple sclerosis, arteriosclerosis and vascular disease can cause damage to the arteries, smooth muscles and fibrous tissues necessary for erection. Diabetes is the biggest culprit, with between 35 to 50 per cent of diabetic men suffering from erectile dysfunction.

Infections

- Penis bugs can temporarily stop his flag from rising. A viral infection of the testes may cause discomfort and also prevent a successful erection. Bacteria can also inflame the urethra and surrounding skin, which can interfere with an erection. Finally, the prostate gland can become inflamed during an infection, which causes a lot of pain in the genital region.

Injuries

- Trauma to the penis, spinal cord, prostate, bladder or pelvis can also lead to ED by damaging the arteries, muscles and tissues of the chambers in the penis. This is not, however, common. In very rare cases, an accident or direct physical injury can be to blame.

Hormone problems

- No matter how romantic the setting, unless he has enough sex hormones, the brain-to-penis transmission won't happen, because he won't be aroused. (It's normal for a man's testosterone levels to decrease with age, but such changes usually happen gradually and don't completely erase the libido.) This is usually caused by the psychological situation (see Mind Games on p.124) rather than a real physical problem.

CURES

Pill PDE 5

- Inhibitors are prescription tablets that help relax the blood vessels in the penis so allowing blood to flow into it, causing an erection. They act within 15 to 25 minutes and can be effective for up to two hours.

Penis injections

● An erection-boosting drug (such as alprostadil) is injected directly into the shaft of the penis, causing stiffening within 15 minutes.

Needle free

● Needle-Free Version: a small pellet of drug, about half the size of a grain of rice, is introduced into the urethra (the tube through which urine is passed) using a special disposable applicator. The pellet is then absorbed through the wall of the urethra and passes into the erectile tissue, giving an erection within 5 to 10 minutes.

Viagra

● See Erection in a Bottle on p.128

Vacuum pumps

● A simple device that works exactly as the name implies, like a vacuum. This is primarily used to treat those with blood disorders, or who use blood thinners.

Hormone treatment

● Men are less likely to have hormonal imbalances that affect their arousal. The most common is low levels of testosterone, which can be bumped up with hormone replacement therapy.

Surgical treatment

● The ED is caused by abnormalities in blood-flow into and out of the penis that can be treated with surgery.

Penile prosthesis

● This is the choice of a desperate man. An implant is generally the last port of call when all else has failed. There are two types: semi-rigid rods and a hydraulic device. The semi-rigid rods maintain the penis is a state of rigidity all the time, but allow the penis to be bent downwards. The hydraulic device is more sophisticated and causes stiffening of the penis when a pump (implanted in the scrotum) is activated.

Therapy

● If the problem psychological, sexual therapy may help.

ERECTION IN A BOTTLE

Viagra has become the treatment of choice for erectile dysfunction, working for two-thirds of the men who try it. The little blue pill does its job by causing the chemical messenger that stimulates erections to persist in his body longer than it normally would. This keeps narrowed blood vessels open thus allowing an erection to occur.

Viagra doesn't produce erections; rather, it sets the stage for them to occur naturally. He still needs some sort of sexual stimulation for one to happen (he usually needs to pop a pill one hour before sex – it's effective for about four hours). Because Viagra works so well, there's a danger of forgetting that it's medication, not a magic trick. And like all medications, it comes with cautions. Any drug containing nitrate, notably nitro-glycerine (used to treat angina symptoms), can be a lethal mix with Viagra.

His erection seems to last forever – too long! What should we do?

Sufferers of the unfortunately termed Retarded Ejaculation (RE) find it difficult to ejaculate. Although they may be fully sexually aroused, and enjoying the stimulation, orgasm seems to take for ever, if indeed it comes at all. Some sufferers of RE have no problem with self-masturbation, but tense up completely with a partner. The cause can be physical or mental – only his doctor can tell for sure.

My new boyfriend can't get an erection. He says it only happens with me and that he gets hard just fine on – ahem – his own. Is it that I don't turn him on?

He isn't being a (soft) prick. Erectile Dysfunction (ED – the new term for impotence) could very well be partner-related, especially if he is getting erect other times. For instance, some men have found they need Viagra when with one woman but not another. Just because his bouts of ED are happening with you doesn't mean it's you who is causing them. The problem is all in his head.

If you're in the middle of things when ED strikes, try this hand manoeuvre to resuscitate him: use your thumb and index finger to create a makeshift cock ring around the base of his penis. Blood flows into the penis through arteries close to the centre of the shaft and then flows out through veins near the surface. The blood can get in, but if the shaft is squeezed, it can't get out as easily, which gets him harder and keeps him that way longer. To bolster a budding erection, maintain the finger ring as much as possible.

His erections are fine until he starts to put a condom on.

Pre-condom stimulation from hand or mouth is a very nice, direct sort of sensation. But once the condom is rolled on, that stimulation stops. He's not a machine that stays on once it's been switched on.

The condom could also be too tight, cutting off his circulation. When the flow of blood to the penis is interrupted, the 'hardness' diminishes. Try one of the larger sizes (but make sure the fit is still snug or he may as well wear a sieve). See Chapter Seven for how to customise your condom and make the condom-entrance part of your sex play.

My boyfriend has had bouts of impotence and is worried it will happen again. Is there any way to prevent impotence?

Erection problems can be mainly physical, mainly psychological, or a tricksy combination. The problem is that a flagging erection tends to be a self-fulfilling prophecy: the more it happens, the more he thinks it will happen and ergo, the more it happens. To break the cycle, he needs to break whatever habit is causing his occasional failure to rise to the occasion. (If his ED tends to be more of a permanent thing, he may have a serious medical condition and needs to be checked out.) Bad habits are often the cause of an occasionally lapsed erection. The problem is, once the problem starts, the more likely it is for him to slip into a permanent slump. Luckily, all it takes are a few lifestyle changes to get him back in his groove again (see Will He Go Limp On You? on p.127).

He can't get it up – what can I do?

Check under the duvet at about three o'clock in the morning. Men normally get hard every ninety minutes during their sleep (called REM erections). If he stays soft all night, he may have a medical problem.

Erections start in the brain, and end up, well, you know where they end up. Arousal happens in the brain, and a chemical reaction allows the muscle that keeps blood from flowing to the penis to relax. Between the brain and the penis, many physical things can happen prevent erections.

What do penis pumps do?

They're marketed for ED. But repeated use supposedly results in the lengthening and thickening of penis. Apparently the suction causes a huge erection and then a strap is wrapped around the base of the penis so it stays engorged. This intense hard-on allegedly stretches the penis muscles, expands capillaries and in 6 to 8 weeks, voila, more man! But don't order one just yet. Because they stretch out the tissue of the penis, after prolonged use a penis pump can cause his penis to become floppy at the base, like it's on a hinge, turning his al dente into limp linguine.

BOOKS

THE SEX-STARVED MARRIAGE: A COUPLE'S GUIDE TO BOOSTING THEIR MARRIAGE LIBIDO
(Simon & Schuster, 2003)
by Michele Weiner-Davis
In contrast to its tabloid title, this book offers candid and sensible counsel for couples with mismatched libidos.

RESURRECTING SEX: SOLVING SEXUAL PROBLEMS AND REVOLUTIONIZING YOUR RELATIONSHIP
(Quill, 2002)
by David Schnarch, PhD
By showing couples how they can turn their worst sex and relationship disasters into personal growth and spiritual connection, Dr. Schnarch offers couples the best sex of their lives.

A PATIENT'S GUIDE TO MALE SEXUAL DYSFUNCTION
(Handbooks in Health Care Company, 2000)
by Tom F. Lue
This pocket-sized consumer text covers what causes erectile dysfunction, finding the cause, treatment options, finding the right doctor, case studies, and a glossary.

FOR WOMEN ONLY: A REVOLUTIONARY GUIDE TO RECLAIMING YOUR SEX LIFE
(Owl Books, 2002)
by Jennifer Berman, Laura Berman and Elisabeth Bumiller
This comprehensive handbook's purpose is to arm women with the information they need about their bodies and sexual responses, and to provide them with the full spectrum of options for treatment for sexual dysfunction.

RELATE GUIDE TO SEX IN LOVING AND RELATIONSHIPS
(Vermilion, 2001)
by Sarah Litvinoff.
Easy to read advice on problems for men and for women, from the leading agency offering couples and sex counselling.

INFORMATION AND ADVICE

The Female Sexual Psychophysiology Laboratory homepage.psy.utexas.edu/homepage/group/MestonLAB/Resources/dysfunction.htm
If sex is painful, then click here for a down-to-earth overview of possible causes, and help, from this UK-based organisation.

The Sexuality Information and Education Council of the United States (SIECUS)
www.siecus.org
This is the place to go for sexuality education, sexual health, and sexual rights information.

The American Association of Sex Educators, Counselors, and Therapists (AASECT)
Email: aasecct@mediaone.net
Website: www.aasect.org
A non-profit organisation that includes sex therapists as well as physicians, nurses, social workers, psychologists, allied health professionals, clergy members, lawyers, sociologists, marriage and family counsellors, family planning specialists and researchers and students in relevant professional disciplines. behavior.

The Society for Sex Therapy and Research (SSTAR)
www.sstarnet.org
This is your one stop shopping center for locating sex educator, counsellor or therapist in your area.

The Society for the Scientific Study of Sexuality (SSSS)
Email: thesociety@inetmail.att.net
Website:www.ssc.wisc.edu/ssss
Dedicated to the advancement of knowledge about sexuality.

International Society for the Study of Women's Sexual Health
Email: isswsh@wjweiser.com
Website: www.isswsh.org
Exists to to provide the public with accurate information about women's sexuality and sexual health.

Relate
www.relate.org.uk
If you live in the UK, contact this organisation to find out about couple and individual psychosexual therapy and how to find a counsellor near you. Relate is the largest single provider of sex therapy in the UK. It is the major trainer of psychosexual therapists and its training is accredited by the British Association for Sexual and Relationship Therapy www.nhsinherts.nhs.uk

www.embarrassingproblems.com
For answers to all your most red-faced sex-related questions.

www.bettydodson.com
You will find out more than you ever knew you needed to know about masturbation here.

Kinsey Institute
www.indiana.edu/~kinsey
You can find out practically every study ever made about sex – and realize that no matter how isolated you feel, you are not alone.

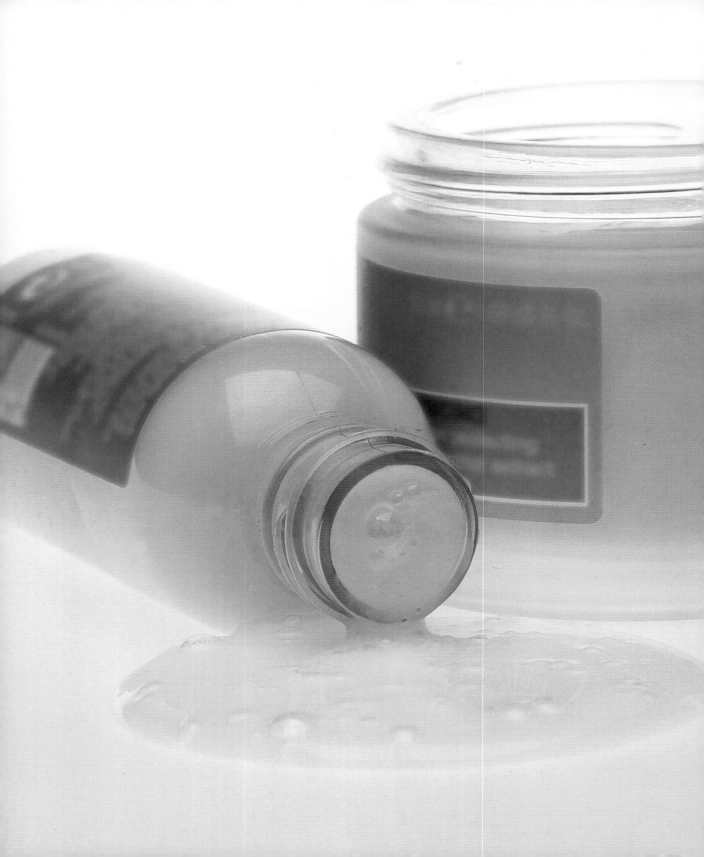

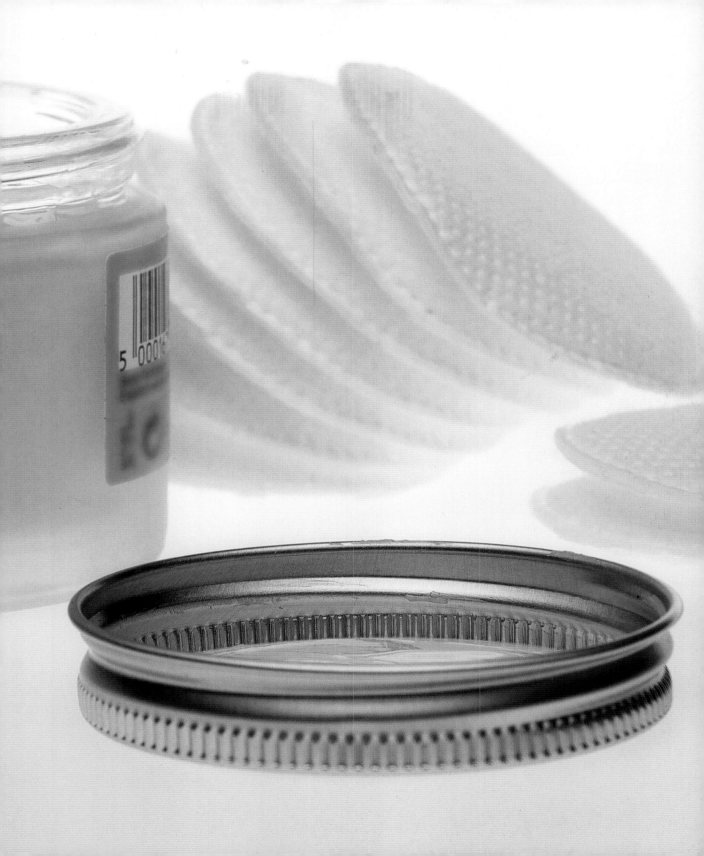

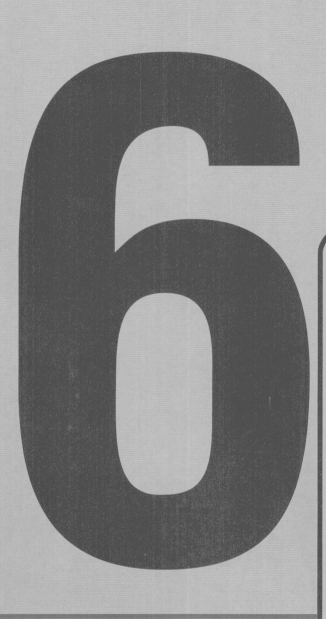

5 Safe Sex Habits

(1) Don't apply too much pressure when you use a vibrator. It can result in tears in the delicate vaginal tissues, causing heavy bleeding and pain.

(2) Silicone water-based lubes are not water soluble, so they don't get absorbed into the skin. This means is they are ultra-slick and slippery and stay that way longer, making them ideal for anal sex as well as water sex.

(3) Watching and waiting is not a good method for figuring out if you've been infected. Just because your vagina hasn't turned green or started disintegrating doesn't mean you're healthy. If you suspect you've been infected, get checked out. Early detection is often the key for cure without complications.

(4) Brushing or flossing your teeth too vigorously may cause cuts or inflammation to your gums or lining of the mouth, or even ulcers. These openings could be a way for STDs to be transmitted during oral sex.

(5) Next to abstinence, using condoms is the best protection against most sexually-transmitted infections.

PLAYING SAFE

Everything you need to know to have safe sex

Pregnancy, STDs, injury, cancer, pain and/or even death are not things we usually think of when we have sex. But all are possible and possibly even probable – depending on how close to the edge of the wild side you lie when it comes to sex.

Yes, everyone wants their sex to be passionate, zipless and spontaneous. However, because of the way that sexuality works in all of us, the more responsible you are, and the more safe and protected you feel, the easier it is to be really aroused and to enjoy sex. Worry and fear about disease, infection and pregnancy can actually inhibit your brain from cranking out arousal messages to your body. That close-down can result in vaginal dryness and tightness. For men, it can mean trouble with erection or premature ejaculation.

RISKY BUSINESS

What is the discharge that drips out of his penis before sex?

Those love drops are called pre-ejaculatory fluid. Think of it as penile lubrication. It helps a man make a smoother entry. Usually a clear, mucus-like substance, the amount varies from penis to penis and from one sexual experience to another.

Pre-ejaculatory fluid may contain some sperm or infect you if he has an STD.

Will it hurt my vagina if he sticks his fingers up?

The vagina is made for penetration and fingers are a lot slimmer than the average erect penis. But just as you don't want to give entry to a dirty penis, his digits should be clean or he may give you a vaginal infection (see Chapter Two). Also, the penis does not have nails – make sure his are well trimmed or you may end up with small tears in your delicate vaginal wall, which could also lead to infection and/or painful sex.

How safe is it if he comes on my hand and then I touch my vagina?

Sperm survive only in a warm, wet environment, and will die within seconds without it. When all of the semen dries, you are not in any danger of impregnating yourself. However, if his ejaculation is still moist when it makes contact with your vagina, there is a possibility of pregnancy, even if you've never had intercourse. If you're ovulating, which is the ideal time for fertilisation, the sperm can potentially move into the vagina and backstroke on up to your egg. And an STD is always a possibility if you have an open cut that comes in contact with his semen.

This guy and I were going at it hard when we both heard a crack. He lost his erection and hasn't been able to get it up since. Did his penis break?

Despite the name, there are no actual bones in his boner. However, he can fracture his member. The penis is composed of tough layers of spongy erectile tissue (which, when aroused, become engorged with blood).

Vigorous sex, especially when you're on top, increases the pressure and can cause a rupture to the works. Usually, this just causes bruising as blood spills out into the surrounding tissues. But about 20 per cent of the time, the urethra can actually be damaged. In which case, bleeding will occur from there. If it isn't repaired, he can develop a chordee (bent penis) or, worse, suffer from erectile dysfunction, in which a leak prevents the penis from trapping blood. Either way, he needs to get to the doctor for a once-over.

Although my boyfriend loves going down on me, he often has a terrible sore throat afterwards. Is that normal?

If you are the only woman he's ever had a sore throat with, then you might have a bacterial bug such as bladder infection (see Chapter Two) or an STD such as chlamydia or gonorrhoea (see Chapter Eight) that is attacking his throat. The only way to know for sure is to get a doctor to do a quick MOT on your vaginal fluids.

Less likely, he may have strep throat, gingivitis, periodontal disease or another infection of the gum and mouth that is making his pipes go dry. He might even have oral herpes, a virus that causes red sores to erupt in the mouth and throat, so he should get checked out for that as well.

> In a rare phenomenon called penis captivus, a man becomes stuck inside a woman when her vaginal muscles suddenly clamp together. The couple remains locked in intercourse until he loses his erection and can slide out.

Sexual First Aid

Sex isn't all fun and games. Here's how to cope with some of the more typical injuries that can crop up in a good night's work:

THE DAMAGE	REMEDY	NEXT TIME...
Rug burn	Smear on antibiotic ointment, then cover so they stay moist until they form a scab.	Climb on top.
Penile fracture	See question on opposite page.	Have him pump less enthusiastically.
Broken skin from a love bite	Wash well – if there's infection (fever, swelling, discharge), you'll need antibiotics.	Give him a hickey and decide if it adds to your love life or not.
Claw marks	Antibiotic ointment	Trim your nails.
Sore penis or vagina	Bed rest (not that kind)	Use your organs more sparingly.

If you both get a clean bill of health, it could be as a result of his technique. He might be so excited by the sight of your vagina (sweetie!) that he pants and heaves, causing soreness. In which case, he can try moistening up by sucking on hard candy during oral sex. Better yet, he can suck on a menthol lozenge, which will soothe his throat and make you tingle. Keep a glass of cool water by your bed for frequent hydration, and try not to knock it over in a frenzy.

Remember, if you are giving him unprotected blow jobs and he has an infection, you are also at risk.

My boyfriend loves it when I milk his prostate. Is it dangerous?

Could be. Because it is situated on the nerve pathway between the penis and the brain, the prostate is an ideally positioned pleasure centre. In fact, it's often called the male G-spot (though it's a lot harder to reach than the female version). As access is only through the anus, massaging it makes it prone to bacterial and viral infections which can cause prostatitis. Here's how to play safely:

● Make sure your nails are short and use a glove to protect him and you from germs (this is his bum hole after all – think about what passes through and then you decide if you want to stick a naked finger in there).
● Use lots and lots of lube.
● The more aroused he is, the more relaxed his back entry will be.
● Go slowly, first rubbing the flesh between his scrotum and anus (the perineum, also known as the love triangle for its erogenous qualities) and the rim around his bottom hole.

● Ease one finger in about three or so inches, finger facing up. The prostate should feel like a walnut-sized lump (bigger if he's older) on the front wall of his rectum. To massage, or 'milk' it, as you say, bring your finger up in a come-hither kind of motion or in a clock or counter clockwise direction move, applying gentle, continuous pressure. Don't poke or forcefully push on it. This can damage the prostate.

● As soon as your finger comes out, take off the glove, throw it away and wash your hands.

> Moving a penis, finger or mouth from one place (such as the vagina) to another (such as the anus) without putting on a new condom increases the risk of moving the infection.

How can I do anal sex safely?

By acting like a good scout: be prepared and take precautions. The problem doesn't come so much from putting the penis in the anus as from thrusting a naked penis in an unlubricated anus, causing small tears, lesions and pain, and exposing the penis and anus to possible (and possibly deadly) infection. So remember your three Ls – lube (lots of it, the water-based kind), love glove and logic – as in, the penis is not a battering ram and should not be used as one.

Is it okay to finger the vagina after using the same finger that has been in the bum?

Only if the digit has been washed and scrubbed to ER standards. A finger that's explored the depths of the anal cavity has picked up some bacteria on its travels. Normally, the urethra and bladder have no bacteria. Bacteria that manage to enter the bladder are usually removed during urination. Without washing, this finger's non-stop trip into the vagina can cause infection, such as a UTI (see Chapter Two). That's why women wipe from front to back, rather than from back to front, after they pee and poo to prevent bacteria from getting into the vaginal area and bladder.

Is it okay to use something other than a finger up the bottom?

It isn't as elastic as the vagina (which, after all, is biologically constructed to let a ten-pound package pass through), through the opening of the anus, or anal sphincter, does stretch – to a point. It can safely accommodate an erect penis, tongue, or just about any slender item. However, objects may be sucked up into the rectum past the sphincter, so hold on tight. And use plenty of lube.

After anal sex, I noticed blood on my boyfriend. He wasn't cut anywhere. Should I be worried?

Hold off on more back door fun until your bleeding has completely gone. Serious injuries from anal sex are relatively rare. Generally, if you see blood or have an internal pain after using your rear entrance, it's:

● A haemorrhoid: this is a swollen vein in the anal area. They're fairly fragile and prone to bleeding (if you have haemorrhoids, you'll feel a swollen, soft fleshy tender lump in the anal area). Treatment is a few tedious steps, but if followed, the haemorrhoid will heal within a few weeks. It involves soaking in a bath with salt for 20 minutes three times a day and analgesic creams and ointments to temporarily numb the pain and provide relief. You can't hold off on bowel movements until your haemorrhoid heals, but over-the-counter stool softeners and a high-fibre diet will keep your things soft and easy to pass.

> Roughly 35% of heterosexuals and 50% of the gay community practise anal sex at least occasionally.

● Anal fissure: this small tear in the lining of the anus can cause pain as well as bleeding. Even mini fissures can be pretty painful, because they often cause spasms of the opening of the anus. They heal slowly because they're irritated repeatedly every time you use your bottom to make a bowel movement. Treatment is the same as with a haemorrhoid.

● Perforation of the colon: basically a hole, this

7 Infections You Can Get Through Back Door

1. Herpes
2. AIDS
3. Hepatitis B
4. Gonorrhoea
5. Syphilis
6. Chlamydia
7. Genital warts

complication can happen after anal sex, but it is pretty rare. If you also have fever, severe pain and pressure on the abdomen, then get medical attention right away. The hole can be repaired with surgery and antibiotics will prevent infection.

If I use my tongue on his bum, am I going to taste poo?

The rectum is just a passageway. The waste is actually stored in the colon, but even if he sterilises the area, you are still likely to encounter only a few stray bits.

Analingus or rimming (the names for anal oral sex) is pretty risky stuff, because it puts the mouth – which is a breeding ground for potentially harmful bacteria – in direct contact with another high-germ area. The partner with the active tongue can get a variety of intestinal parasites (causing fever, cramping, and diarrhoea). Then there's also viruses like herpes, gonorrhoea, HPV and hepatitis on the STD front (see Chapter Eight). Similarly, there's the possibility of open cuts or tears in the anus which can expose you to blood infected with HIV. While a good wash can help 'freshen' the anal opening before analingus, it will not necessarily rid the area of germs.

SAFETY RULES

I recently had a one-night stand with a guy I don't know and will never see again. We didn't use protection. What now?

First, kill your chances of pregnancy with emergency contraception (see Chapter Seven). Then get tested for STDs. And tested again. And again. STDs have a wide range of incubation periods. While chlamydia can show up within two weeks of infection, HIV can take up to six months to appear.

Here's what you'll need to do to get tested for the seven most common STDs: get a physical exam for genital warts (shows up anywhere within three weeks and eight months of contact) and herpes (generally within one to three weeks). Get your cervix, urethra and/or bum swabbed for trichomoniasis (give it four to 20 days), chlamydia (symptoms appear between one

Over 90% of cases of cystitis (see Chapter Two) are caused by E.coli.

5 Bum Rules

1. Use lots of lube. When in doubt use more rather than less.
2. Go slowly. Allow the anus time to adjust and get used to whatever you place in it.
3. The rectum is lined with thin sensitive tissue that tears easily. Make sure nails are trimmed, all jewellery has been removed and any toys used have no sharp or rough edges or ridges.
4. Use a condom or finger glove (on toys as well).
5. Clean anything – fingers, penis, toys – that has been up the bum very well with soap and water before using it again.

and three weeks), gonorrhoea (symptoms will show within ten days) and a blood test for hepatitis B (you can get this immediately after contact) and HIV (you may need to wait at least six months).

While you're waiting for that second round of tests, pay careful attention to your private parts. Watch for symptoms like white or flesh-coloured warts (signs of genital warts), angry red blisters (possible herpes), and painful peeing (possible chlamydia). If you notice any strange sensations, lumps or bumps, tell your doctor ASAP.

Needless to say, next time you go flinging, get him to don a sheath.

I'm tired of waking up next to a guy I barely know and wondering if he's given me some disease.

So don't do 'it', but do everything else. Most sex consists of brief, genitally focused foreplay, intercourse, orgasm and sleep. That's not to say that this sort of bread-and-butter intercourse is offensive or that it doesn't feel good. But it is anticlimactic for a woman since her pleasure centre is located outside the vagina (the clitoris, see Chapter Four).

Outercourse is lovemaking without penetration into a vagina or an anus. No semen, vaginal fluids, or blood is shared between partners. So it gives you all of the pluses of sex (orgasms, the excitement of holding back, freedom from guilt and regret) and none of the minuses (fear of pregnancy and most STDs; weird mornings – after you realise that you've opened yourself completely to a guy you know almost nothing about).

> Wear a latex or polyurethane condom each and every time you do the deed – from now until you settle down with one mutually monogamous partner. Safe sex is the best way to prevent passing on most STDs that you may have contracted. It's also the best way to avoid catching most of them from future partners.

This is not a flashback to fifties-style petting and cuddling. Here are your five steps to ecstasy, keeping your clothes (mostly) on (individually or combined, they can all result in orgasm):

- Making out: Kiss, kiss and kiss some more.
- Body rubbing: The couple rub their bodies over each other's with abandon.
- Masturbation: You'll learn what each other likes without the usual fumblings and worries.
- Mutual masturbation: Continue to do the above, except do it to each other.
- Blowing: Oral sex is not considered 100 per cent safe unless protection – a condom or dental dam (see Chapter Seven) is used.

> Chronic anal fissures may require surgery. Doctors commonly perform two procedures to ease the tension around the wound, allowing it to heal shut. The first procedure is anal dilation, involving stretching the anal canal. The second is internal lateral sphincterotomy, which requires removal of part of the anal canal musculature.

It's just not exciting to stop a guy to make sure he wears a condom.

And pregnancy and STDs are exciting? The thinking is, 'Here comes the latex, and there goes the spontaneity'. Not so! The key is to make putting the condom on erotic so you don't lose the erotic momentum.

When is it safe to lose the latex?

After you've checked all of the following. You've both been:

- Monogamous (only with each other physically – and yes, kissing, oral sex, mutual masturbation and anal sex are all included in that package – for one year and are planning to keep things status quo).
- Practising safe sex without exception for the entirety of that year;
- Tested twice, six months apart, during that year, for all STDs and tested negatively for all.

8 Reasons Not To Leap Into Bed

(1) You don't want to and that's a good enough reason! You don't have to have sex, full stop – not ever, not anywhere and not with anyone, if that's your choice. You can be celibate for as long as you want and it's nobody's business if you are. Thanks but no thanks works well.

(2) He'll never call again unless you get it on. Oh really? A man who actually says that is an insensitive idiot and therefore not your type, right?

(3) You think he'll never call again unless... Well he may not be an insensitive idiot but clearly you think he is. Why have sex with someone you have a low opinion of?

(4) You just found out he cheated. He's apologised and wants kiss-and-make-up sex. Make sure he's made his way up to a genito-urinary clinic (GUM) and been tested for STDs.

(5) Neither of you has a condom. No birth control, no nookie, unless you've talked seriously about having babies together before tonight.

(6) You can't decide whether he's exciting or scary. Exciting = good. Scary = not so good. Can't tell the difference? Then wait, all will be revealed. And then you can either sleep with him or run for your life.

(7) You have an active herpes sore or HPV wart or any STD that is currently contagious – or he does (see Chapter Eight). Love does not mean sharing everything.

(8) It makes a nice change.

Is it possible to have too much sex?

Frequent sex has been associated with cervical cancer (see Chapter Two). However, it is pretty well accepted that cervical cancer can be caused by genital warts. People who have indiscriminate, unprotected sex are at a higher risk for such STDs. So it may be the fact that they have risky rather than frequent sex. Or it may be a combination of the two. There are people who have a lot of sex without any health problems because they are careful about whom they sleep with, take the proper precautions, and get regular check-ups. These are good habits everyone should have.

The longest kiss ever lasted 417 hours.

Bottom line: there is no definitive if-you-go-over-this-then-you're-sick number of times for doing the deed. So, as long as you're doing it safely, your body isn't feeling too tender, you're not neglecting the rest of your life for a constant roll in the hay, you're still eating and sleeping and involved with things other than sex, then enjoy yourself.

SEXESSORIZE

Are all sex toys safe?

Stay away from sharp objects, spiky things and anything that looks like it might hurt. Also think about the material: soft silicone, latex or rubber is more comfortable than hard plastic or metal. And use as intended – butt plugs do not belong up the vagina.

Is it safe to put syrup or any type of stuff down there during oral sex?

Most things are fine as long as you're not using latex (condoms, diaphragms, cervical cap). Then you have to make sure your additive doesn't contain oil, which can eat a hole in latex.

Is there a herbal sex-booster that works?

Herbal cures are seldom backed by the rigorous research typically found behind mainstream drugs. However, some herbs are at least safe and possibly helpful in dealing with sexual problems. See p.144 for what to look for (and avoid) when doing it au naturel.

5 Potentially Deadly Bedroom Risks Women Take

(1) RISK You always use a condom – except for that ten per cent of the time when you don't.
REALITY CHECK One of the leading cause of death for 25- to 44-year olds worldwide is AIDS.

(2) RISK You think one of the following:
1. 'I know him, so it's okay.'
2. 'If he withdraws before ejaculation, it's okay.'
3. 'If it's only oral sex, it's okay.'
REALITY CHECK Knowing someone does not make unprotected sex any safer than having a casual danger fling – the only way to know for sure is if he has recently tested negative for most STDs (however, some STDs have a long incubation period and tests will get false-negative results).

(3) RISK You had unprotected sex and it was okay, so you figure it's okay to do it again.

REALITY CHECK Every time you have unprotected sex, your chances of catching an STD go up.

(4) RISK You asked the crucial questions:
1. How many partners do you have in one month?
2. Did you have safe sex?
3. Have you had an STD?
4. Have you had an HIV test?
5. What were the results?
REALITY CHECK Good questions, but think – have you ever lied about how many partners you've had? Studies show that 96 per cent of women and 92 per cent of men lie about their past sexual history to current partners.

(5) RISK Telling him to use a condom doesn't fit with your image as a freewheeling sex goddess.
REALITY CHECK Does death?

SEX TOY MAINTENANCE

Increase the life of your sex toys

- Never dunk your vibrator in water, unless it is specifically sold as a waterproof vibrator.
- Clean your toys after each use by rubbing with something like surgical spirit and a clean cloth.
- If your toy has a power cord, don't pull or bend the cord very much. No matter how well built the toy is, eventually you will break off the cord.
- For the most part, any sex toy sold including batteries will most likely come with cheap ones that won't last very long, and do run the risk of leakage. Toss them out and install some with an established brand name.
- Don't share your toys.
- Silicone dildos and plugs can be boiled for up to three minutes, cleaned with a bleach solution, or run through your dishwasher. For more delicate polymers stick to warm water and soap, and replace them every so often, as they are impossible to keep perfectly clean.

Scream machines for good vibrations

- Vibrators should not be used to directly stimulate the opening to the urethra as it could set off a bladder infection.
- Numbness is not sexy – don't overstimulate your genitals with a vibrator.
- If your vibrator is too powerful, calm the vibrations by placing a towel or cloth over the vibrator.
- Vibrators are not a ladies-only toy. A man can run a vibrator up and down the shaft of his penis, he can use it on his nipples, he can insert it in his butt for prostate stimulation.
- A vibrator is not supposed to be used like a faux penis or a dildo. Most women use vibrators for external stimulation, on their clitoris and outer vulvas, and never use them internally at all.

On hole-makers

- Petroleum jelly
- Chocolate syrup
- Butter
- Hand lotion
- Baby oil
- Massage oil
- Suntan cream or oil
- Thrush antifungal medication
- Vaginal lubricants containing mineral oil
- Talc powder

Love potions

THE INGREDIENT	THE CLAIM	LOVE POTION OR POISON?	PROCEED WITH CAUTION
Yohimbe (comes from the bark of West Africa's Yohimbe tree)	Dilates blood vessels, allowing more erection-nourishing blood to reach the penis.	Possibly a potion	Decide if harder erections are worth elevated blood pressure, irritability, nausea and vomiting.
Ginseng	Encourages the body to make testosterone and increases sperm production.	Potion – if it contains the designation Panax (which means it's of American or oriental origin) and contains 15% ginsenosides.	Insomnia, raised blood pressure, headaches, irritability
Royal jelly	More potency	Poison	Can cause asthma attacks, severe allergic reactions and death.
St John's Wort	Can boost libido	Potion – if it is 600–900mg of a 0.3% standardised extract.	Can work against the Pill, making it ineffective.
L-arginine	Causes better blood flow to the genitals.	Taking up to 1,000mg may give it potion qualities.	Waste of money
Damiana or wild yam	Sexual stimulant	Poison	Waste of money
Chocolate	Sexual stimulant	Minor potion – it contains a stimulant which creates feelings of excitement.	Oh, the calories and fat!
Ginko	Widens blood vessels of the genitals.	Poison	Avoid if you have heart problems.

Are 'Brazilian' bikini waxes safe?

Before you dare to go bare, take heed: a Brazilian wax removes all of your pubic hair, except for a thin vertical strip front and centre, and all the hair around your vaginal lips and anus is removed. In other words, ripe for an infection (particularly folliculitis, an infection of the hair follicle that causes it to become red, tender, and filled with pus, spread rapidly to other follicles and require treatment with antibiotics). Less frequent side effects are superficial skin burns from improperly heated wax, and rashes in reaction to chemicals.

> If he doesn't want to de-pierce, thicker latex condoms can act as a shield against his armour and ease any irritation that you may be experiencing. Look for condoms that don't advertise 'thinner' on the box.

To avoid a wax gone wrong, go to a clean, reputable spa where the waxings are performed by licensed aestheticians who wear latex gloves, use disposable wooden sticks to apply the wax and work in sterile settings. Even so, once there, make sure your skin is cleansed by an antiseptic before and after waxing, so that bacteria on the skin's surface cannot get into the open hair follicles. Also make sure your aesthetician doesn't double dip the spatula into the wax. Once it touches your body, it's time to break out a new one. And beware industrial-size batches of wax. You don't want the goo to have been cooking for weeks.

Is it safe to dye my pubic hair?

Those who choose to colour below the belt do so at their own risk. The reason is that the major companies that manufacture hair colour only test their products on head hair. Therefore, they can only ensure that their products are safe when used as directed.

If you're determined to go ahead, only colour the hair that covers the mons pubis (the soft area of fatty tissue over the pubic bone). Avoid the hair on the labia (lips of the vulva), where the dye will probably cause severe irritation. It's also important to avoid getting the product in or near the vaginal lining or mucous membrane. The equivalent danger zones for men are the shaft of the penis and scrotum.

Gels and creams, including products used for men's beards and moustaches, may work better for thicker hair. They are less likely to drip and may provide better control in the genital area.

> # HOW MUCH OF A RISK-TAKER ARE YOU?
>
> Do you engage in any of the following?
>
> - Anal sex
> - Sadomasochism (S-M or S&M)
> - Sex without a condom
> - Sex outside
> - Sex during your period
> - Getting pierced on your genitals
> - Bondage
>
> The more 'yes' answers you have, the more you have the odds stacked against you. Which may seem sexy, spontaneous and daring, but it can also be dangerous. So if you're going to take risks – and obviously you are – then you should know the facts.

> Skip the cock ring at the airport as it could be caught by the metal detector.

Even though I clean it, my tongue piercing still flares up. What's amiss?

Piercings anywhere other than your ears invite infection. So keep superclean. Don't pick at it, wash twice a day with antibacterial soap, don't overlube the area with lotions or oils, and try to avoid tight threads.

Nature lovers

Three scientifically-proven health reasons to do it outside:

- Sunlight is nature's: Viagra. One theory on why sunshine seems to kick-start sex drive is that it suppresses melatonin, the hormone believed to be the biological version of a cold shower. Sunshine is also thought to rev up serotonin and other hormones that makes us more open to beach blanket bingo.
- His mini-me rises with the heat. There's evidence that testosterone skyrockets when it's between 65 and 85 degrees outside. In fact, studies have found that men who live in tropical regions may have higher testosterone levels than those living in cooler climes.
- Your nose knows. Your sense of smell improves in hot weather, so it's easier to sniff out your partner's pheromones, basically the come-hither scents our bodies put out when they want a little nookie.

A basic kinktionary

Auto-erotic asphyxiation: choking to orgasm supposedly intensifies sensations. That's because the lack of blood flow and oxygen can produce giddiness, lightheadedness, or exhilaration. It's estimated that 30 per cent of all adolescent male hangings are the result of autoerotic asphyxiation.

BDSM: the B stands for bondage, the D for dominance, the S and the M for sadomasochism. Bondage involves sexual play with ropes and restraints. Dominance (and its partner, submission) is a term which is part of power play, in which partners take roles with one being dominant, the 'top' or in charge, and the other submissive, the 'bottom' or a subservient slave. Sadomasochism is a derivation of both sadism, the term which describes a desire for giving another physical pain, and masochism, the sensation of enjoying receiving that pain.

Fetish: a psychological term which refers to an inanimate object which stimulates sexual desire, such as a shoe, a baby bottle, underwear or any other object.

Golden Showers: when one person pees on another for sexual gratification.

Are pierced clits dangerous?

A pierced clitoris is said to intensify sensitivity and pleasure. As far as the procedure is concerned, the hood of the clitoris is more commonly pierced than the clitoris itself – the process is less complicated and therefore safer. It takes the skin approximately one to two months to heal after the piercing is done. You then must clean your piercing twice a day with an antiseptic solution to prevent infection.

My new boyfriend has a pierced penis. Can it scratch me down there?

It depends on his fashion sense. If he's into a small, smooth hoop, you're probably okay and his dick jewellery might even make sex more of a turn-on. However, if he is sporting a stud, it may cut you up a bit. Earrings with rough edges can cause lots of cuts so small that they can't be seen and cuts may lead to infection.

That said, the vagina is pretty good at protecting itself, because regular sex will cause some small abrasions, too. So it's unlikely that anything will happen. Just be sure to keep a lookout for bloody discharges after sex.

> An estimated 95% of paraphiliacs – that's fetishists, voyeurists, paedophiles and those with other sexual disorders – are men.

Nature's Safe Sex Spoilers

DOING IT AT THE:	WATCH OUT FOR:	ANTIDOTE
Beach	Wet bathing suits create the perfect environment for thrush (see Chapter Two).	Change ASAP
Any green area	Stinging nettles	Antihistamines may help take the sting out of a rash.
On the ground	Biting insects	Apply anti-itch cream.

Are cock rings dangerous?

As long as he doesn't leave it on 24/7, it's fine. A cock ring is most often used to make an erect penis harder and bigger, to keep it that way for a greater length of time and to delay and heighten orgasm. They're slipped over the shaft and the testicles/scrotum when the penis is soft. The cock ring will constrict blood flow, keeping blood in the shaft of the penis. When a wearer finally does ejaculate, the sensation is more intense, since it took a longer time to come, and because the penis is filled with additional blood. The ring bearer should wear it for no more than 30 minutes maximum. If he crashes out with it on, the blood could be trapped for hours, which can damage the delicate blood vessels in his penis.

It seems like doing it in water is cleaner and therefore safer – yes?

Try no. Whether good old H2O (bathwater, say), salt water or chemical-laden pools or hot tubs, the water is going to wash away your own wetness, creating irritation and sometimes infection. What's more, condoms are a tricky affair in the deep. Water could get under the rubber, causing slippage, or chlorine and chemicals from pools and such could weaken the bag, possibly causing breakage (so much for a fun splash-about). And in a hot tub, exposure to high temperatures may damage latex, leaving you open to STDs and/or pregnancy.

Also, soaking in a hot tub causes blood vessels to dilate so his erection may not be as firm. Dilation of the blood vessels also cause dizziness or a headache, especially with exertion. Maybe you should stick to the bedroom.

If you are going to do it in water use silicone-based lube to assuage dryness, enter before you submerge and, once in the water, keep your thrusts to a minimum, if possible.

Is kinky sex safe?

Yes, as long as you establish rules before you start the games. To most people these days, 'kinky' involves some degree of sadomasochism (S-M). Mutual consent is what distinguishes (S-M) from abuse and assault, just as consent distinguishes sex from rape. And one woman's kinky may be another's turn-off, so be clear about 'stop and go signals' for both parties.

PROTECT YOURSELF

I've heard a lot about date rape drugs. What can I do to check my drinks?

- Party by the buddy system. Check in with friends every 20 minutes. If something seems strange, leave immediately.
- Watch for signs of over-intoxication. If you are leaving the party, let your friends know where you are going and with whom.
- Designate someone to be the sober 'lookout' – someone who can drive and can keep an eye on things.
- Do not accept drinks from anyone other than a bartender or waitress. Always open your own drinks if they are offered by someone else.
- Do not accept drinks from a punch bowl or other open container.
- Never leave your drink unattended. If you go to the bathroom, take it with you. If you get up to dance, finish it or take it with you. A friend left to watch your drink can easily get distracted.
- Don't drink anything that has a funny smell, colour or taste. If it seems strange, throw it out right away.

5 Questions That Can Be Answered In One Word

(1) In how many minutes do most women reach orgasm using a vibrator?
Three

(2) Genophobia is a fear of... what?
Sex

(3) What percentage of people are aroused by S & M?
10

(4) Which gender tends to take more risks?
Men

(5) Which gender tends to be more at risk from unsafe sex?
Women

I was raped a few years ago. I am still having difficulty with my sex life. I get aroused, but I am never able to reach orgasm. What can I do?

Rape is a terrible violation of your body and probably of your trust in men. Rape survivors often have difficulty with consensual sex, even with someone they love. Intercourse may have come to be associated not with pleasure and intimacy, but with the fear and humiliation you suffered during the assault.

These feelings can show themselves in a number of ways. You may tense up, not allowing yourself to relax or to achieve orgasm. You may 'disassociate' or remove yourself mentally from the situation. Or you may avoid sex altogether, out of fear that it will call up troubling emotions or even flashbacks to the event itself.

Having sex in a meaningful relationship is one way to be able to relax and trust your lover. Telling your partner what happened to you also means that you can work with him on ways he can help you feel comfortable during sex. One rape counsellor technique recommends that if you start to freeze up, he should say something like, 'It's OK, it's me, you're safe now.' Or if you begin to disassociate or 'space out,' he can say, 'Talk to me, tell me what you're feeling right at the moment.'

You should work out these responses beforehand, so that they don't remind you in any way of the rape. There are things you can do, too, to feel less threatened. You may want to practise achieving orgasm on your own, stimulating yourself in a safe, familiar place: the bathtub, your own bed.

When you do have sex with your partner, notice and focus on physical differences between him and the man who attacked you, or between the location where you were raped and the place you are in now.

If you feel a flashback coming on, replace it with a calming image – a waterfall, a beach, any vision that soothes and reassures you.

Also, consider therapy. Talking over your fears and feelings with an empathetic listener can only help.

> Many rape victims experience "flashbacks" – getting intimate with someone (whether it be the first time or the fifty-seventh) makes you flash back and remember things or feel feelings you may have bottled up because it reminds you of the rape act.

What should I do if I am raped?

If, despite your best efforts, the worst happens, it's easy to go into a daze or into denial. But you need to take action ASAP. Even if you decide you do not want to press charges, you will still need to protect your health. Here is your six-step plan:

- Go to or contact a friend or family member you can trust, who can be with you indefinitely and immediately (if you think you've been drugged, you need to be tested).
- As much as you will want to, don't take a shower until after you contact the police and are tested. Showering can remove important evidence like semen, skin and hair, and clothing fibres.
- Try to recall details of the event and of your attacker (hair/skin colour, height/weight, clothing, scars and tattoos, etc), any vehicle and its details (state, licence plate, make, model, colour, dents), location, or anything else, and write these down.
- Call the police or go with someone you trust to a station to report the rape. State as soon as possible that you wish to prosecute. This will initiate the testing you will need and better reporting of the incident. You can change your mind later. (Remember, alcohol abuse does not legally justify anyone's behaviour, and cannot be used as an excuse in a court of law.) All police stations have specially trained staff who deal specifically with victims of sexual violence. Many police stations have a special location where victims of any kind of sexual crime can be interviewed. It is usually either a house or a set of rooms designed to help put the victim at ease. There is usually an examination room and a bathroom with a plentiful supply of hot water and clean towels, where you can bathe after the forensic examination.
- Seek medical attention as soon as possible after you have been tested. You may have internal injuries you're not aware of, so the sooner you get examined, the better.
- Talk to someone trained in rape counselling to begin your healing.

BOOKS

THE ULTIMATE GUIDE TO ANAL SEX FOR
WOMEN
(Cleis Press,)
by Tristan Taormino
This book covers a topic that the author knows
in depth on a personal level. It is factually
accurate and conveys all the information the
readers might need while managing to capture
the pleasure and passion which the author finds
in her chosen subject.

INFORMATION AND ADVICE

Sex Boutiques
In general, the more reputable the company, the better the product and the info on how to use it. Most ship worldwide, using discreet brown wrapping.

Ann Summers
www.annsummers.com
There are stores throughout the UK plus a website. Also a source of hosting sex toy parties.

Blowfish
www.blowfish.com
The hip sex toy shop with a good section of toys, books, and videos.

Good Vibrations
www.goodvibrations.com
One of the founding sex toy shops in the US. Retail stores in San Francisco and Berkeley, California.

Libida
www.libida.com
Geared toward women with a good range of toys, books, and videos reviewed by its female staff and good solid advice on how to choose a product.

LoveHoney
www.lovehoney.co.uk
A wide selection of goodies.

Sh!
A women-friendly shop in the UK run by women.
www.sh-womenstore.com

Xandria
www.xandria.com
A company geared mainly for couples.

www.sexuality.org/l/incoming/aanal.html
Log on to this website to get the insider info on anal sex.

www.sexual-health-resource.org/anal_sex.htm
Covers everything you need to know about anal sex, including the advantages, disadvantages, hygiene, history, gay anal sex, risks and methods.

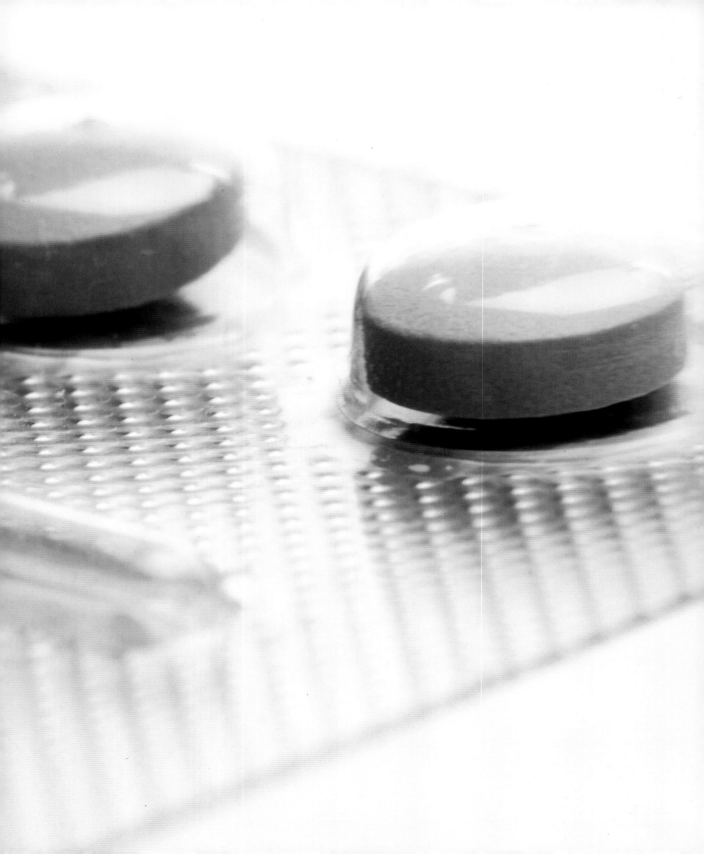

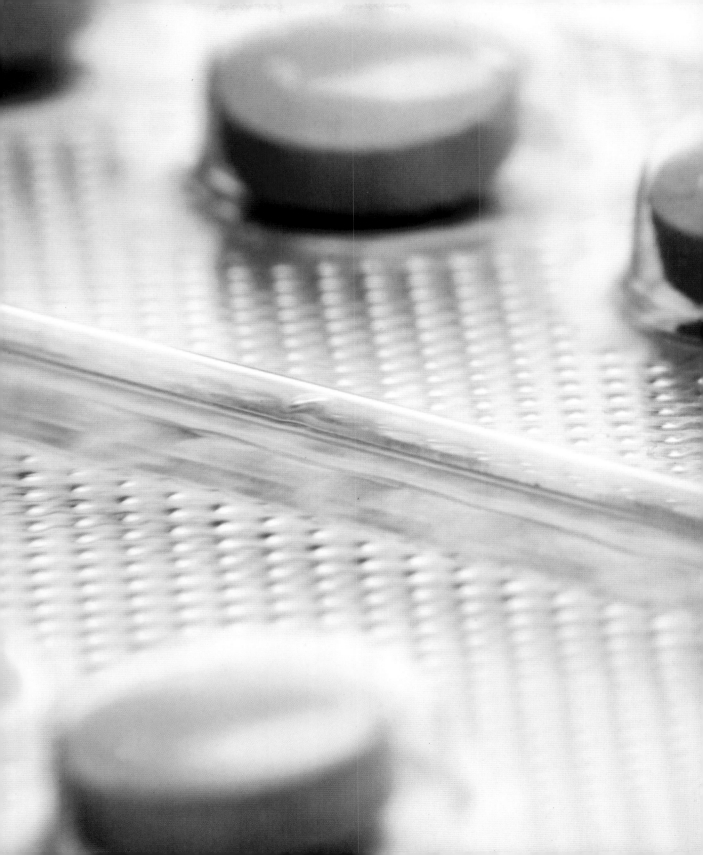

7

5 Healthy Contraceptive Habits

(1) Choose a birth control that fits your needs. If you have a busy, hectic lifestyle, birth control you are required to think about daily, such as oral contraceptives, may not be the best option.

(2) Don't have sex under the influence. Drug or alcohol use can impair your judgement and your motor function significantly.

(3) Reassess your method when: you change sexual partners, settle down with one partner, before and after pregnancy, during and at the end of nursing, when you have a medical disorder diagnosed, when a new method becomes available, when your family is complete.

(4) Remember, pregnancy affects your body more than his. Take responsibility for making sure you are always protected when you have sex. Don't leave contraception up to chance or your lover.

(5) Remember, the kind of contraception you choose can affect your chances of getting an STD.

ARE YOU A PREGNANCY WAITING TO HAPPEN?

Everything you need to know about contraception, getting pregnant, and abortion

Here's a surprise. The typical woman who uses contraceptives other than sterilisation can expect to get pregnant by accident once in her lifetime. That's because even the most effective birth control methods fail occasionally, and because perfectly diligent birth control users are hard to find.

Consider the Pill: it's 99.9 per cent effective when used precisely as directed. In the real world, however, five out of 100 Pill users get pregnant in the first year of use. Multiply that over 10 or 20 years, and you can see that even good methods used over long periods can result in a fair number of pregnancies.

The most effective form of birth control is the one that works best for you. Each form of contraception comes with its own set of pluses and minuses. Some have side effects you would rather live without, such as vaginal dryness, weight gain, higher risk of UTIs. Others hinder the sexual lifestyle you envision for yourself – you want to be able to have regular sex on the spur of the moment without worrying about putting something on or in.

TAKE YOUR PILL

How long does it take for the Pill to take effect?

Longer than you'd like. Your first packet of birth control pills probably won't give you the same level of protection against pregnancy as the following months' pill packets will (assuming they are taken correctly). The reason is, there's a chance of an egg being released before you take the first Pill. Most birth control pills rely on the action of the hormone oestrogen, which essentially inhibits the release of an egg from the ovary.

Combination pills that contain oestrogen and progestin (a synthetic version of the hormone progesterone) might provide a little more protection in the first few weeks. This is because progestin works a little differently from oestrogen. It is believed that progestin decreases the ability of sperm to penetrate the cervical mucus (in order to swim through the uterus and fallopian tubes to fertilise an egg) and prevents the lining of the uterus from developing normally, so that a fertilised egg would find it difficult to implant in the uterus.

Regardless of the type of birth control pill you are taking, it is always recommended to use a back-up method of birth control, such as a condom, diaphragm, or cervical cap, until you've completed your first pill packet. It's also a good idea to keep a back-up method of birth control on hand in case of emergency (see Oops! on p.164)

I've heard the Pill causes cancer.

Today's Pill contains only about one-fifth of the oestrogen and one-tenth of the progestogen of the early pills; this is more than enough to prevent pregnancy, but far less risky. So many of the hazards associated with the older version, including blood clots, cancer and heart disease, are absent from newer formulations. In fact, the Pill can actually boost your health. (See 14 Reasons You Should Start Pill Popping Right Now on p.160)

That's not to say, however, that taking birth control pills is as harmless as drinking bottled water. Women with certain health conditions such as high blood pressure do face certain risks (see Is Your Birth Control The Best For You? on p.174). And even the healthiest women can have nausea, mid-cycle bleeding or mood changes on these lower dosages.

I want to go on the Pill, but I don't want to gain a single pound.

You don't have to. Most women typically put on about four pounds in the first three months of going on the Pill because the oestrogen it contains can encourage sodium and water retention in your body and can also turbocharge your appetite.

However, there are low-dose formulas of the Pill that contain a type of progestogen that acts as a diuretic so there's no bloating. Ergo, no weight gain. Other pluses: fewer mood swings, less spotting and breast tenderness.

I recently broke up with my boyfriend, so I stopped taking the Pill. It's been a month and I still haven't got my period. Is this normal?

Completely. It takes a while for your ovaries to get back on track so you may end up waiting a week, two weeks, a month or miss your first 'non-pill' period completely. Depending on the woman you are, the type of pill, the length of time you have been taking it and how regular your periods were before you were on the Pill, it may even be a year or longer before you need to buy a box of tampons.

I think I have been on the Pill for too long.

Studies show the longer, the better:

- After one month, you're half as likely to develop PID (see Chapter Eight). The Pill's hormone progestogen thickens bacteria-blocking mucus in the uterus.
- After six months, blemishes vanish in at least 75 per cent of cases.
- After one year, your risk of endometrial cancer (see

DO YOU KNOW
YOUR CONTRACEPTIVES?

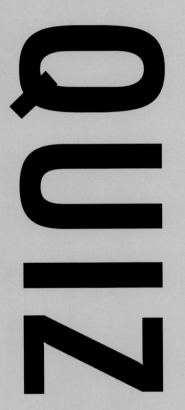

QUESTIONS

① Which method provides protection against STDs?
a Condom, b Sponge, c Oral contraceptives, d IUS, e Spermicide

② How many times a year should you take the following:
- Oral Contraceptives
- IUS
- Hormonal Injection
- Hormonal Implant
- Birth Control Skin Patch

a 40, b For up to five years, c 280
d Once, e Up to 6.5

③ EC (emergency contraception) must be taken within how many hours?
a 24, b 36, c 72, d 120

④ Which will decrease the effectiveness of oral contraceptives?
a Forgetting to take it, b Taking it a few hours late, c Having thrush, d All of the above

⑤ Rhythm Method and Withdrawal Method are the same types of birth control. True or False?

ANSWERS

1 (a) Condom. Other than abstinence, consistent and correct use of latex or polyurethane condoms can significantly reduce the risk of STDs. But remember, STDs can be transmitted through any activity that involves skin-to-skin contact, including vaginal or anal sex, oral sex and heavy petting.

2 Oral contraceptives/280. IUS/once. Hormonal Injection/For up to 6.5. Hormonal Implant/For up to five years. Birth Control Skin Patch/40.

3 The correct answer is both **(b)** and **(d)**. This as a trick question. The IUS can be inserted five days after unprotected sex, ECs must be given with 72 hours of the incident.

4 All of them – **(a)**, **(b)**, **(c)** and **(d)**.

5 False. In the 'rhythm method', women track their periods and temperature changes during the cycle to determine when they are fertile. With the withdrawal method, the couple may have penile-vaginal intercourse until ejaculation is impending, at which time the man withdraws keeping all semen away from the vagina.

14 Reasons You Should Start Pill Popping Right Now

(1) Helps your fertility, part one. The Pill's hormones may inhibit two problem-causing conditions: PID (see Chapter Eight) and endometriosis (see Chapter Three).

(2) Helps your fertility, part two. Studies have found that the longer a woman is on the Pill, the more likely she is to conceive quickly when she does try to get pregnant. The reason may be that by preventing ovulation, the Pill actually may keep ovaries 'younger'.

(3) Lowers cancer risk. Taking the Pill can protect you against ovarian cancer (see Chapter Two), one of the most deadly cancers affecting women, and endometrial cancer (see Chapter Two), the most common cancer of the reproductive system. It may also inhibit another killer – colorectal cancer. Neither current nor former takers of birth control pills are at increased risk of developing breast cancer.

(4) Prevents benign breast cysts. Up to 90 per cent of patients see improvement in the symptoms of fibrocystic breast conditions (see Chapter One).

(5) Treats endometriosis. While progestogen-only oral contraceptives are an effective treatment, the side effects are numerous: irregular bleeding, fluid retention, and depression have made this option unbearable for many women.

(6) Banishes functional ovarian cysts. Oral contraceptives may help prevent these cysts (see Chapter Two) by helping to regulate the menstrual cycle.

(7) Limits PCOS symptoms. (see Chapter Three). The Pill stabilises or helps up to 50 per cent of PCOS-related excess hair growth.

(8) Tames periods. The steady flow of oestrogen and progestogen helps regulate your menstrual cycle so your periods come like clockwork, menstrual flow is lighter, and cramps are minimised or eliminated. With reduced blood loss each month, women on the Pill are also less likely to experience iron-deficiency anaemia, which affects up to 20 per cent of women.

(9) Banishes PMS. That regular supply of hormones also may eliminate many PMS symptoms such as bloating and breast tenderness.

(10) Clears up skin. Oral contraceptives reduce androgen hormones, excessive amounts of which have been found to cause spotty skin.

(11) Makes you sing. Several controlled studies have found that, compared with non-users, women on the Pill report better moods – not just during the premenstrual phase but all month long.

(12) Makes you want to do it. Pill users have reported more frequent and more satisfying sex than non-users. Possible reasons: lighter menstrual periods, reduced PMS, and the spontaneity the contraceptive allows.

(13) Helps you age gracefully. As women enter their mid-30s, their ovaries begin a slow process of shutting down, producing oestrogen more erratically. As oestrogen levels rise and fall, women notice heavier, longer periods, more PMS-like mood swings, and even occasional hot flushes. This is called perimenopause, and its symptoms become more pronounced as women enter their 40s. By keeping women's oestrogen levels on an even keel, the Pill minimises those symptoms. The Pill's oestrogen may even delay or prevent bone loss.

(14) Can be used as an emergency contraceptive. See Oops on p.164

Chapter Two) drops by 40 per cent (progestogen is thought to help protect against the cancer).

- After eight years, you cut your risk of the deadly colorectal cancer (which includes cancer of the colon, rectum, anus, and appendix) by 40 per cent.
- After five years, you're half as likely to develop ovarian cancer (see Chapter Two). After ten years, 80 per cent less likely. Suppressing ovulation may prevent cancerous cell growth. That protection can extend for 15 years or more after Pill use ends.

BURN RUBBER

The condom keeps slipping off my boyfriend. Is it too big for him?

Quite a few things could cause him to slip:

- The condom is too big (see Customise Your Condom on p.162).
- Too much lubricant inside the condom before it's put on. Put a little less in there, or go without lube altogether.
- Vaginal dryness (commonly experienced by women on Depo-Provera) could cause a pulling effect on the condom as you and your partner make love.
- It could be your position, especially if you've noticed that the condom escapes only when you and your partner are in a love clinch.
- Erections can come and go, causing the condom to loosen its grip and slip off. A smaller-sized condom, or saying and doing things that will maintain arousal during sex, may help.

Which are the best and worst condoms?

There are over 100 different kinds of condoms on the market – some so wonderful you want to wear them yourself, others you wouldn't wish on anyone. But it's all very personal. Here's what to look for in general when choosing your party hat; after that, you're on your own:

- Only condoms marked with the Kite mark, CE mark or BS3704 seal of approval are safe and effective.
- Choose your material:

- Latex condoms will protect you from pregnancy and most STDs. They come lubricated, unlubricated and with spermicides. They tend to have a rubberised odour.
- Polyurethane condoms will also protect you from pregnancy and most STDs. They are thinner than and twice as strong as latex, and they are odourless and flavourless. They also transmit heat better than latex and are more resistant to heat and light damage. In addition, they do not have the proteins in latex condoms that cause allergic reactions in some people. However, they aren't as elastic as latex, so the breakage factor is higher. They're also more expensive and do not come unlubricated.
- Lambskin will protect you from pregnancy but not STDs.
- Most condoms come lubricated and include a spermicide, usually nonoxynol-9.
- Condoms also come ribbed and nubbed and coloured and flavoured. Generally, the flavoured condoms are for oral sex only and don't give as much protection for intercourse (after all, it's not like your vagina has taste buds). Texture is a matter of personal preference – some people claim the bumps and ridges enhance pleasure, others claim they can't feel a thing.
- Condoms also come in a variety of sizes (see a Customise Your Condom on p.162). However, you can have a condom with all the bells on and it is still only going to be as good as its operator.

> Women who weigh more than 11 stone need a higher dose of the Pill because the average amount of the Pill's active ingredient, ethinyl estradiol (EE) is stored in body fat – the more body fat, the less EE circulates, making the user 60 per cent more likely to get pregnant.

CUSTOMISE YOUR CONDOM

It used to be that one size fitted all. But studies found that while the diameter of most condoms is 5 cms (2 in), one-third of all penises are wider than that. Enter the customised condom: regular, snug or large. Regular will fit most men. The snug fit or contoured condoms are meant for Slim Jims and measure slightly less across. Finally, large size, meant for the XXLs, come in two varieties, roomier around the head and bigger all around.

The best way to find his fit is to use the toilet-paper-roll test. Slip an empty tube around his pecker when it's fully awake. If it fits like it was made for him, he's like 90 per cent of guys and needs a regular-size raincoat. If there's room for stretching, he should use a snugger fit. And if you're stuffing him in like a Christmas goose, he needs to go up a size.

What's the difference between a male and female condom.

Here's what's similar: Both work as a barrier method of contraception (i.e. they block sperm and infection from entering your vagina).

My boyfriend puts on a condom just before he's about to penetrate me, but it always makes him lose his erection. Is there a better time to do it?

There's only one time: as his penis stands up to attention. The moment a guy starts feeling arousal, his penis can start dripping with pre-ejaculatory fluid. While the risk is pretty low, if that fluid comes in contact with your vagina, you could end up pregnant or, if he has an STD, infected.

If his penis gets soft after you've gloved him up (see Chapter Five for more on why this happens), you'll need to chuck the old condom and start all over again, even though he hasn't ejaculated in it. That goes even if he only loses his erection for a minute, as the condom could leak.

To keep him hard, try putting the condom on him yourself. Press the flesh between his scrotum and anus. This is a guy hot spot and the pressure may be enough to keep him hard while you suit him up.

It seems that no matter what type of condom my boyfriend and I use, they always burn me. What's wrong?

It sounds like you have an allergy – not to your boyfriend and not to sex, but to latex condoms or the spermicide that's on them.

Latex, a milky fluid produced by the rubber tree, is used to make condoms, balloons, rubber bands, tyres, washing-up gloves and medical supplies such as IV tubes and syringes.

In some people, latex can trigger an allergic reaction that leads to a red rash that itches and burns. In extreme cases, it can even cause an asthma-like reaction: nasal congestion, a runny nose, shortness of breath, and wheezing.

> Hold onto the condom before pulling out. This way, he'll leave your snug room fully dressed.

Condoms are often lubricated with nonoxynol-9, a spermicide that can also irritate sensitive skin. Because it acts like a detergent, it can create microscopic sores or tears that burn or sting during sex.

About two per cent of people are sensitive to latex, while about ten per cent are sensitive to nonoxynol-9. Try condoms that have no spermicide and are made from polyurethane. These are just as effective at preventing STDs and pregnancy as regular latex condoms.

Male Or Female

MALE CONDOM	FEMALE CONDOM
It's an outie – it fits over an erect penis.	It's an innie – it is inserted into the vagina.
The failure rate is three per cent with perfect use and from 14 per cent to 16 per cent with typical use.	The failure rate is five per cent with perfect use and 21 per cent with typical use (possibly because users may not have the hang of inserting it yet).
He needs to have a full erection before putting it on and is put on right before penetration.	It can be put on up to eight hours before the party starts and he doesn't have to pull out as soon as he's left a deposit.
Comes in latex and polyurethane.	Comes in polyurethane (thinner but stronger than latex).
Strong and silent type.	The baggy shape lends it to making 'vart-like' noises during use.

I bought a packet of condoms several years ago. Can I still use them?

It depends on what kind they are. Look at the expiration date printed on the package. Condoms with spermicide have a three-year shelf life (if kept in a cool, dry place). After that, the spermicide isn't active, although the latex is still reliable. Plain latex condoms expire five years after manufacturing, because the latex becomes less resilient and prone to breaking after that much time has elapsed. An old condom is better than no condom, but why risk it? If they've expired, they should be retired.

GOING NAKED

I want to use natural contraception but I'm not sure how to figure out my cycle.

Women tend to ovulate mid-cycle. However, it is more accurate to say that they ovulate 14 days before menstruation (see Chapter Three). Women have been known to ovulate at any time during their cycle, including during menstruation, although this is generally quite unusual.

In terms of conception, fertility depends on three factors: a healthy egg, healthy sperm, and favourable cervical mucus. A woman ovulates once a cycle. The egg lives 12 to 24 hours and then disintegrates if not fertilised. Under favourable cervical mucus conditions (cervical mucus nourishes and guides the sperm, which would otherwise die in about a half an hour or never reach the egg), sperm can survive five days in the body.

So if you want to use ovulation prediction as birth control, you can't just avoid sex on the day you ovulate (you'll notice more clear vaginal lubrication – it'll look and feel like egg whites). You've got to stop the contraceptionless hankie-pankie at least five days before the egg comes down the hatch (and charting

HOW TO PUT ON A CONDOM SO IT DOESN'T BREAK, TEAR OR SLIP

It's not enough to use a condom. You have to use it correctly. Approximately two to five per cent of condoms tear during use. The majority of these failures are caused by dumb human error. Here's your total coverage insurance:

- Test drive different condom brands to help him find the one that fits most comfortably (see Customise Your Condom on p.162).
- Make sure the condom has passed testing and isn't past its expiration date.
- Never store the condom in a warm place, as it weakens the latex.
- Lose the accessories: rings or long, sharp, or jagged fingernails can create microscopic tears in the latex.
- Don't skimp on foreplay – a lack of lube during sex intensifies friction which ups condom slide-off risks
- Slip the condom on when he's fully erect but before he's leaking pre-ejaculate juices.

Follow these five simple steps to avoid the usual mistakes people make when suiting up:

- Put a dab of water-based lubrication on the tip of his penis before to smooth things along (anything oil-based will erode the latex).
- Don't unroll the condom before you put it on. Instead, place it over the head of the penis and unroll to the base while…
- Pinching the tip to force out any air as you unroll the sheath to the base of his penis. This will also create empty air space – a place for the semen to go (lack of doing this is cause number one for breaks).
- Once the condom is on, you can take the extra precaution of smoothing out any air bubbles (number two cause for breaks).
- Don't linger – the condom can leak if he withdraws after he has shrunk from ejaculating (cause number three). Hold the rim of the condom down along the base of the penis when removing the penis after ejaculation.

your cycle is the only way to figure out when the unsafe times starts). Of course, if you want to get pregnant, just do what comes naturally around that glorious ovulation day.

If you have good sex, then it's one more reason to play it safe and use birth control. Your orgasmic contractions can help suck the sperm up the vaginal canal, bringing them closer to your egg. One study found that if a woman climaxed any time between one minute before to 45 minutes after her partner ejaculated, she ended up with much more sperm in her vagina (and therefore a higher chance of pregnancy).

OOPS!

I lost a Pill down the sink.

Usually, if you miss a Pill, you should pop it when you remember and take the next Pill at its scheduled time, even if it means downing two Pills in one day. If you're less than three hours late, just resume your schedule.

If you're more than three hours late you will have to abstain from sex or buy condoms to use until your next period, because you will not be protected from pregnancy. If you get your period as scheduled, start the next Pill cycle as normal.

He wore the condom inside out. What are my chances of pregnancy?

Very low, as long as you didn't take it off and flip it around. Using a condom backwards is not uncommon – the biggest risk is the condom tearing because it is inside out. Problems start when you realise that it's inside out and flip it around. If your naked vagina comes into contact with any pre-ejaculatory fluids that may already be on what is now the outside of the condom, you could be at risk of pregnancy and STDs.

Help! The condom broke!

Luckily, there is one thing you can do that will reduce your chance of pregnancy by as much as 90 per cent. Get your doctor to prescribe Emergency Contraception (EC – see Break Open In Case of An Emergency on p.168). This treatment blocks pregnancy, but it is NOT the same thing as an abortion, which terminates pregnancy. What EC can't do is prevent disease, so wash your vagina with mild soap and water but don't douche.

Unfortunately, it's a waiting game when it comes to STDs (up to six months for an HIV test; even genital warts can take a year to show). Mainly, it's a balance of paying attention to any changes in your body (heavy vaginal discharge, nausea, temperature – see Chapter Eight for more symptom information), without obsessing over every little pelvic ache.

It's a good idea to stock up with a spare packet of the Pill, just in case you lose one.

I forgot to get my Depo-Provera shot. What are my chances of getting pregnant?

Pregnancy is rare for most women who are between two and four weeks late getting their next shot, but it still can happen. Some doctors will administer a shot at up to four weeks late, but that's pretty much the limit. Start using a condom or some other form of back-up until you get your next shot.

8 Times You Don't Have To Worry About Getting Pregnant

1. When you are already pregnant.
2. When want to get pregnant.
3. When you're using your birth control correctly (see Common Contraception Cock-Ups on p.166 and How To Put On A Condom So It Doesn't Break, Tear or Slip, opposite).
4. When one of you has been surgically sterilised, or is infertile.
5. When you are having safer 'outercourse' rather than intercourse.
6. When you are having anal or oral sex.
7. When you are practising abstinence.
8. On the day you ovulate.

Fertility Advice You Can Ignore

1. Drinking coffee.
2. Taking an over-the-counter cough preparation that contains guaifenesin, which has a thinning effect on cervical mucus that is purported to help sperm swim through the reproductive tract.
3. Keeping him out of close-fitting, polyester-lined underwear.
4. Giving up strenuous exercise.

Common Contraception Cock-ups

(see Is Your Birth Control The Best For You on p.172)

BIRTH CONTROL	COCK-UP	THE FIX
Latex (condoms, diaphragm, cap)	Adding oil – it eats holes in your latex, too tiny to see, but big enough to let in sperm. There is oil in lipstick, chapstick, hand and face creams, butter, petroleum jelly, vitamin E and ointments for rashes and sores (e.g. those for thrush, herpes or haemorrhoids). Lotions that say water-soluble are not water-based, so they could still contain oil that eats latex.	Read the label carefully.
Condoms	Using two at once as erection protector or double safety insurance can make them rip. The friction between the two condoms, can make them tear or slip off.	One used correctly is as safe as it gets (see How To Put On A Condom So It Doesn't Break, Tear Or Slip on p.164).
The Pill	Ignoring sick days: 1. Antibiotics, anticonvulsants, tranquilisers and antifungals lessen the Pill's effectiveness because they cause the liver to break down the hormones in the Pill faster than normal. 2. If you vomit within an hour or have diarrhoea within four hours of swallowing your Pill, there's a chance the hormones will not have been completely absorbed. 3. St John's Wort can weaken the potency of the Pill by about 50 per cent.	1. Take the Pill, but use a condom while on antibiotics and continue for seven days after. 2. Some doctors suggest inserting the Pill vaginally as an alternative to missing a Pill if you're suffering from nausea, and/or vomiting. 3. Talk to your doctor about all medications you are taking, including alternative ones.

BIRTH CONTROL	COCK-UP	THE FIX
Implanon	Certain drugs used to control epilepsy and TB, as well as some antidepressants and barbiturates, can tamper with this method's pregnancy-blocking hormones.	Switch to another birth control method if you use these drugs.
Spermicidal inserts	Thrush medications have active ingredients that can reduce the effectiveness of nonoxynol-9, the chemical used to kill sperm.	Use another method while using the medication.
Diaphragm	Not getting resized regularly. Weight gain or loss or pregnancy (even if you don't carry the baby to term or you have a caesarean) can change the shape of the vagina and pelvic tissue, affecting the fit of the diaphragm.	Get refitted any time your body weight fluctuates by more than ten pounds.

BREAK OPEN IN CASE OF AN EMERGENCY

- The condom broke or slipped.
- Your diaphragm or cervical cap moved out of position.
- You had sex without using a contraceptive.
- You missed your regular contraceptive shot.
- You missed two or more Pills in a row.
- You were forced to have sex.

You have two ways to practise pregnancy damage control when contraception fails:

Plan one: EC Pills are high-dose birth control pills containing oestrogen as well as progestogen. EC pills work much like birth control pills. They can stop or delay ovulation (the release of an egg), prevent sperm from fertilising an egg you've already ovulated, and stop a fertilised egg from implanting in the uterus. It does not stop a pregnancy that has already started. They must be taken within 72 hours of unprotected sex (followed by a second dose 12 hours later), so you can't procrastinate and just 'wait and see what happens'. However, the sooner you use it, the more effective it is.

You can get emergency contraception from:
- Any GP who provides contraceptive services.
- Any family planning clinic.
- Any young people's or Brook clinic.
- Most genito-urinary (GUM/sexual health) clinics.
- Some hospital accident and emergency departments (phone first).
- Some privately run clinics, including the British Pregnancy Advisory Service (BPAS).
- Most NHS walk-in centres (England only).
- Some pharmacies.

Plan two: Have your doctor insert an intrauterine device (IUS). You can do this up to five days after unprotected sex (see, Is Your Birth Control The Best For You? on p.174).

PREGNANCY INSURANCE

I'm 28. Should I worry now about having a baby in five years?

Don't ignore the clock. If you try to get pregnant at age 21, the odds are about 60 per cent that you'll be looking for nappies during any given month, but your chances drop to about 25 per cent by age 35. Women are born with their eggs already in one basket: about one million of them to be precise. And those eggs have a shelf life. By puberty, you only have about 300,000. As you get older, you have fewer high-quality eggs, which increases your risk of having a baby with a chromosomal abnormality such as Down's Syndrome.

There's no need to panic yet, but you may not want to wait ten years to start trying to get pregnant. At age 35 about three-quarters of women will eventually be able to conceive without medical treatment, but by age 40 only half will. By age 45, it's under 10 per cent.

I have irregular periods: does that mean I'm infertile?

If you have a cycle that is very long (more than 36 days) or short (less than 22 days), it's possible that your ovaries aren't functioning normally, and that could impact on your eggs when you try to get pregnant. Every woman's cycle is different. Before you start budgeting for infertility treatments, see your doctor to rule out possible medical causes for your erratic cycle. Weight swings, thyroid disease, endometriosis, Polycystic Ovary Syndrome and fibroids can interfere with your cycle (and possibly your fertility).

Termination Choices

TYPE	Medical (AKA abortion pill)	Vacuum aspiration abortion
AVAILABILITY	Only in the first nine weeks of pregnancy	
HOW IT WORKS	Two abortion drugs: 1) Mifepristone (sometimes called Mifegyne or RU486). Blocks the action of the hormone that makes the lining of the womb hold onto the fertilised egg. 2) Prostaglandin. Given 48 hours later, this causes the uterus to cramp. The lining of the uterus breaks down and the embryo is lost in the bleeding that follows. The pain has usually settled within six hours or so.	A thin, round-ended plastic tube is eased into the uterus through the cervix. Using a gentle pump, the contents of the uterus are passed into the tube. You may experience some discomfort, similar to strong period pains, because the uterus usually cramps during the process. The procedure takes 10 to 15 minutes, with a total clinic stay of up to two hours. (Under general anaesthetic, the procedure is slightly different and you'll need to stay at the clinic three hours.
PLUSES	Anaesthesia is not required, no surgical instruments are used, the experience may resemble a natural miscarriage.	Over quickly, generally requires that women make two visits to a health care provider. Side effects are similar to a normal period.
MINUSES	The bleeding lasts a few weeks, and you may see the foetus when it aborts from your body, side effects can include nausea, headache, weakness, cramping and fatigue. From 1 to 12 per cent of medical abortions fail – which means surgical procedures are required to end the pregnancy.	Requires the use of invasive instruments, and cannot normally be performed in very early stages of pregnancy. Less effective after seven weeks of pregnancy, bleeding lasts at only a few days.

DO YOU KNOW WHAT YOUR CHANCES OF
GETTING PREGNANT

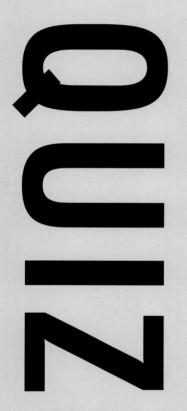

QUESTIONS

(1) What proportion of couples experience infertility?
a 1 in 5
b 1 in 10
c 1 in 20
d 1 in 30

(2) Which of the following is the most usual reason a man is infertile?
a Low sperm count.
b Poor sperm motility.
c Abnormally shaped sperm.
d Some combination of all three.

(3) Match the egg number to the age span:
● 4 months before you're born
● Birth
● Puberty
a 300,000 eggs
b 2 million
c 7 million eggs

(4) For every egg ovulated by the time you're in your 20s, it's estimated that up to 100 are lost along the way. True or False?

(5) All of the following are causes of infertility, except which one:
a A large number of sexual partners.
b Prior abdominal operations.
c Chlamydia (if untreated).
d A prior diagnosis of pelvic inflammatory disease.
e Douching.
f Age.
g Caffeine.

ANSWERS

1 (b) One in ten couples experience infertility at some point during their lifetimes.

2 (d) A combination of factors usually contribute to infertility.

3 4 months before you're born **(c)**, Birth **(b)**, Puberty **(a)**

4 False – 1,000 eggs are lost.

5 (g) Caffeine.

Lifestyle Factors that May Affect Your Chances of Conceiving

FERTILITY SLAYER	WEAPON	PROTECT YOURSELF
STDs	The problem with STDs is that they can spread. Infections that begin in the vagina (such as chlamydia) can move into the higher uterine tract, leading to PID which in turn can quickly lead to infertility (see Chapter Eight).	Use condoms, limit your sex partners (and choose them carefully), visit your gynaecologist and, because many STDs don't come with clear symptoms, ask to be tested.
Smoking	Exposing eggs to nicotine affects their quality – and decreases the ovaries' supply. Smoking also damages the cilia, which move the sperm and eggs through the fallopian tubes. The more cigarettes a woman smokes daily, the lower her chances of conception. Smoking may also speed up the onset of menopause, prematurely closing your lifetime window of fertility.	Quitting now can restore much of your fertility within several months.
Being seriously over- or under-weight	If a woman has too much body fat, the body produces too much oestrogen and begins to react as if it is on birth control. A woman with too little body fat can't produce enough oestrogen and her reproductive cycle begins to shut down.	If your period becomes irregular and your body weight has changed, you need to see your doctor for nutrition and dietary information.
Ageing	Older eggs have trouble conceiving.	You can't stop the clock, but take care of the other factors and you'll keep the odds in your favour.

PREGNANCY SCARE

Ten things you can stop worrying about if you've been caught off-guard by pregnancy:

Contraception

During those few weeks before you realize you're pregnancy, you might have continued to use the Pill or spermicides. Chemicals in spermicides and hormones in birth control pills seem to pose little risk. (The warnings on the labels of birth control pills are pretty dire, but the actual incidence of birth defects is very low.) IUSs pose more of a problem and may increase the risk of miscarriage or ectopic pregnancy. Luckily, it's extremely rare to become pregnant using an IUS, but if it happens to you, call your doctor ASAP.

Medications

Once a pregnancy is confirmed, all medication that a woman takes should be approved by her obstetrician. Only a handful of drugs have been specifically approved for use during pregnancy, chiefly because the research on their safety hasn't been done on pregnant women:

- Aspirin is considered risky because it may cause bleeding problems, although a couple of aspirin early in a pregnancy are unlikely to cause harm.

- While women are advised against using decongestant drugs for colds and allergies during pregnancy because they can decrease blood flow to the uterus, if you've used one of these drugs a few times early in pregnancy, there's no cause for panic.

- A few antibiotics may pose a risk: Tetracycline, for example, may cause a permanent yellowing of baby teeth (if taken after the twentieth week of pregnancy). Streptomycin has been associated with hearing impairment in infants exposed during pregnancy.

- One of the riskiest medications is the drug Accutane, a prescription drug to treat severe cystic acne, because it contains a substance that causes birth defects.

Vitamins

While you want to be on top of your vitamin intake when you're pregnant, one to avoid is Vitamin A, which can cause severe birth defects when taken in large doses (the recommended daily allowance for vitamin A is 2,700 IU per day).

Smoking

The damage can be lethal. Children whose mothers smoked in the early weeks of pregnancy take in less air and so less oxygen. Smokers also give birth to low-birth weight babies. Quitting ASAP can help.

Environmental and Chemical Toxins

These are things like asbestos, paint fumes, mothballs or hair dye – with most of these, one-time exposures pose no serious risk.

Hot Tubs and Saunas

Minimal exposure is fine – if you've had more, talk to your doctor.

Alcohol

As long as you're a sensible social drinker, there is probably very little danger. The risks come from high doses of alcohol consumed in short amounts of time.

X-ray

Unless this is how you spend all your leisure time, there is very little risk from common diagnostic procedures like dental X-rays, mammograms and X-rays of the chest, arms, legs or head, because modern machinery uses very low doses of radiation, and early in pregnancy the uterus is protected by the pelvic bones. Even X-rays of the back or pelvis are probably safe. Only be concerned if you are receiving regular high-dose radiation therapy for cancer.

Caffeine

There is no definite evidence that drinking caffeine is in any way related to problems in pregnancy.

Parasites

Raw meat, raw fish, unpasteurised cheese and (used) cat litter: raw meats and cat faeces can carry a parasite that causes toxoplasmosis, which can lead to foetal abnormalities or toxoplasmosis-associated injuries in young children who were apparently normal at birth. If you were exposed to either of these things early in your pregnancy and experienced a flu-like illness, inform your obstetrician (some women are immune). Doctors recommend that pregnant women refrain from eating raw or very rare fish because it may carry parasites that pose a risk to the mother's health (for instance, tapeworm can cause anaemia). Chances are if you had sushi recently, you're fine but you should tell your doctor. Unpasteurised cheese can contain listeria, which can cause miscarriage soon after it has been digested.

IS YOUR BIRTH CONTROL THE BEST FOR YOU?

Cervical Cap

Thimble-shaped rubber cap you fill with spermicide and fit over cervix.

HOW IT WORKS Prevents sperm entering uterus.

PROTECTION 48 hours.

BABY-PROOFING ABILITIES 84 per cent. Some protection against pelvic inflammatory disease (PID).

SIDE EFFECTS YOU NEED TO KNOW ABOUT May dislodge during vigorous intercourse; it can't be used during your period.

DOES IT RUIN THE MOMENT? No. It can be inserted up to six hours before sex and stay in place for up to 24 hours.

HASSLE FACTOR Medium. Insertion can be a little awkward and the cap must be kept in place at least six hours after intercourse.

PLEASURE BAROMETER None

BAD HABIT PENALTIES Using any oils, as they can cause holes in the rubber.

OPERATING INSTRUCTIONS Before inserting, check for holes or tears by holding it up to the light. Fill one-third to one-half of cap with spermicidal jelly or cream. Insert by squeezing the cap between thumb and index finger, sliding it into your vagina and pressing rim around cervix (feel around the edge to be sure the cervix is completely covered). To remove, press on the rim until the seal on cervix is broken, tilt cap, then hook fingers under the rim and pull sideways out of vagina. After use, wash with mild soap and water, and dry thoroughly; store in a cool, dry, dark place.

DIY? No, you need to be fitted and the fit needs to be checked annually.

MOST COMMON COCK-UP Putting it in incorrectly.

Condom (male)

Latex, polyurethane or animal tissue balloon-shaped cover placed over erect penis.

HOW IT WORKS It bags sperm so it doesn't enter your body.

PROTECTION Instant.

BABY-PROOFING ABILITIES 98 per cent.

STD-PROTECTION 97 per cent (with latex or polyurethane, but lambskin offers no protection) against all STDs except genital warts, herpes and crabs.

SIDE EFFECTS YOU NEED TO KNOW ABOUT Some women have an allergy to latex or nonoxynol-9 spermicide, with which many condoms are lubricated.

CAN IT RUIN THE MOMENT? Yes.

HASSLE FACTOR Low. Can't be put it on until he's hard, must be removed immediately after ejaculation or it may leak.

PLEASURE BAROMETER Condoms help slow down premature ejaculation, they also come in different textures to increase stimulation for you and him. Some men feel their sensations are reduced.

BAD HABIT PENALTIES If the condom is latex, using any oils as they can cause holes in the rubber.

OPERATING INSTRUCTION Keep handling to a minimum. Blowing up the condom to check for leaks, opening the package with your teeth or fingernails and/or stretching the condom can cause tiny tears. If it doesn't unroll, it's on wrong. Start again with a new one. (see How To Put On A Condom So it Doesn't Break, Tear Or Slip on p.162).

DIY? Yes.

MOST COMMON COCK-UP Putting it on too early or late so you don't get a proper fit or tearing it when you put it on/take it off. Also, using with ANY oily extra – like vaginal creams, thrush creams (even if applied a few days before), Vaseline, baby oil and massage oils – breaks down the latex, making it ineffective.

Condom (female)

Shaped like an upside-down sock, it's a larger polyurethane version of the male condom with an inner ring which sits over the cervix and an outer ring which lies flat against the labia (vaginal lips).

HOW IT WORKS Cling films the vagina and cervix, preventing any contact with sperm.

PROTECTION 24 hours.
BABY-PROOFING ABILITIES 97 per cent.
STD-PROTECTION 97 per cent, except genital warts, herpes and crabs.
SIDE EFFECTS YOU NEED TO KNOW ABOUT None.
CAN IT RUIN THE MOMENT? It can be put in up to eight hours before sex.
HASSLE FACTOR High. Putting it on is complicated and you have to remove it right after sex. Also, the outer ring can slip inside you during sex.
PLEASURE BAROMETER Some people feel less sensation because it covers the whole genital area.
BAD HABIT PENALTIES Protection is reduced if you don't remove it once you have sex.
OPERATING INSTRUCTIONS Carefully remove the condom from the package. Hold the condom with the open end down. Use the thumb and middle finger to squeeze the flexible ring at the closed end into a narrow oval. With your other hand, spread the lips of your vagina. Insert the ring and sheath into the vagina. Use your index finger to push the ring as far as possible into the vagina. Insert a finger into the condom until it touches the bottom of the ring. Push the ring up past the pubic bone. Make sure the outer ring and part of the sheath are outside the vagina over the vulva. To remove, spread the lips of your vagina with one hand and reach in with the other to grasp the ring between thumb and middle or index finger and carefully draw out. Throw the condom away.
DIY? Yes.
MOST COMMON COCK-UP Putting it on incorrectly, allowing sperm to leak in.

Diaphragm
A shallow cup you fill with spermicidal cream or jelly and insert up to six hours before sex.
HOW IT WORKS Prevents sperm entering uterus.
PROTECTION 24 hours.
BABY-PROOFING ABILITIES 90 per cent.
STD-PROTECTION Some protection against PID, chlamydia, gonorrhoea and trichomoniasis. It reduces risk of cervical cancer.

SIDE EFFECTS YOU NEED TO KNOW ABOUT It's been associated with urinary tract infections.
CAN IT RUIN THE MOMENT? It can be inserted up to six hours before sex, but you have to add more cream/jelly each and every time he ejaculates (which in itself can be pretty sticky, messy stuff).
HASSLE FACTOR Medium. It takes practice to put in. Then you have to refuel after use, regularly check for holes and get it refitted if you gain/lose a lot of weight. Also, it must be left in place six hours after ejaculation.
PLEASURE BAROMETER Some women say the rim stimulates their cervix.
BAD HABIT PENALTIES Using any oily products (like Vaseline, baby oil and massage oils) are a no-no as they can make your rubber cup leaky. Not adding more spermicide reduces its protection.
OPERATING INSTRUCTIONS Before inserting, check for holes or tears by holding it up to the light. Then spread spermicidal jelly or cream on the inside portion of the dome and rim with clean, washed hands. Put the diaphragm all the way back against the cervix with the cavity containing the spermicide covering the cervical opening; feel around the edge to be sure the cervix is completely covered. If you have sex more than an hour after inserting a diaphragm, or if you have sex more than once in one night, you'll need to squirt some more spermicide into your vagina (don't remove the diaphragm). Leave it in place for at least six hours after his last ejaculation, but no more than 24 hours. Remove it by sticking your fingers into your vagina and gently grasping the rim and pulling. Then wash it with soap and water, dry it, and store it in a cool, dry, dark place.
DIY? No. It needs to be fitted by a doctor or nurse and the fit needs to be checked annually.
MOST COMMON COCK-UP Forgetting to add more spermicide.

Hormonal Implants (implanon or jadelle)
A matchstick-size rod (Implanon) or two rods (Jadelle) containing progestogen, inserted into the arm.
HOW IT WORKS The progestogen is released into

your bloodstream gradually, causing ovulation to stop.

PROTECTION Up to three years (Implanon) or five years (Jadelle). An implant will usually be put in on the first day of your period. You will be immediately protected against becoming pregnant. (If the implant is put in on any other day you will not be protected against pregnancy for the first seven days.)

BABY-PROOFING ABILITIES 99.6 per cent.

STD-PROTECTION Some protection against PID.

SIDE EFFECTS YOU NEED TO KNOW ABOUT Irregular periods for the first year, headaches, acne, weight gain, tender breasts, bloating, ovarian cysts (see Chapter Two).

CAN IT RUIN THE MOMENT? No.

HASSLE FACTOR Low. You'll need an annual check-up.

PLEASURE BAROMETER None.

BAD HABIT PENALTIES None.

OPERATING INSTRUCTIONS The clinician will numb a small area of the arm you use least with a painkiller and then make one small cut to insert the rods. The whole thing takes about ten minutes and is totally painless. Avoid heavy lifting for a few days after insertion. You'll need a follow-up visit within the first three months to make sure there are no problems. The implants must be removed after three/five years when it stops working (you can get it removed earlier if you want). Removal is much like insertion. You can also get restocked when the rods are removed.

DIY? No, the implants need to be inserted and removed by a doctor or nurse.

MOST COMMON COCK-UP Forgetting to have it removed/renewed after three/five years.

Hormonal Injections

An injection of synthetic progestogen in your bottom or arm every three months (Depo-Provera) or every 8 weeks (Noristerat).

HOW IT WORKS The hormone seeps into your bloodstream gradually, causing ovulation to stop.

PROTECTION Three months, starting from day one if you get the shot during the first five days of your period. (If you have the injection on any other day you

will not be protected for the first seven days.)

BABY-PROOFING ABILITIES 99.8 per cent.

STD-PROTECTION Some protection against PID and it lowers the risk of uterine cancer.

SIDE EFFECTS YOU NEED TO KNOW ABOUT Weight gain, headaches, irregular bleeding, headaches and moodiness, and it can take up to 18 months for your body to get back to normal once you stop injections. On the plus side, it reduces period cramps.

CAN IT RUIN THE MOMENT? No. You get the injection and forget about it until the next injection.

HASSLE FACTOR Medium. You need to get reinjected and the injection cannot be removed from your body if you don't like the side effects.

PLEASURE BAROMETER None.

BAD HABIT PENALTIES None.

OPERATING INSTRUCTIONS A shot in the arm or bottom.

DIY? No, you'll need to get an injection.

MOST COMMON COCK-UP Forgetting to get your tri-monthly shot.

Intrauterine Contraceptive Device (IUCD)

A small plastic and copper device that is fitted into your womb. It has one or two soft threads on the end. These thin threads come through the opening at the neck of your womb (cervix) into the top of your vagina.

HOW IT WORKS Stops sperm reaching an egg. It may also make the egg move more slowly along the fallopian tube and/or stop the egg from settling in the womb.

PROTECTION Immediately upon insertion, lasting three to ten years, depending on type (although you can have it removed earlier).

BABY-PROOFING ABILITIES 99 per cent.

STD-PROTECTION None.

SIDE EFFECTS YOU NEED TO KNOW ABOUT Periods may be heavier, longer or more painful. You may have some slight bleeding between your first two or three periods after you have had the IUCD fitted. There is also a possibility of you getting an infection during the first 20 days after an IUCD is put in. If you feel unwell and have any pain in your lower abdomen, with a high temperature or a smelly discharge from your vagina in the first three weeks after the IUcD is fitted, see a doctor as soon as possible. This is because you may have an infection.

CAN IT RUIN THE MOMENT? No.

HASSLE FACTOR Medium. You need to look for the IUcD threads monthly, as it can be pushed out by your womb or can move. This is more likely soon after it has been put in and you may not know it has happened. You will also need to have your IUcD checked four to six weeks after it is put in, and then once a year.

PLEASURE BAROMETER None.

BAD HABIT PENALTIES You can't use an IUCD if you have an untreated STD, have now or have had in the past: an ectopic pregnancy; heavy and painful periods; any problems with your womb or cervix.

OPERATING INSTRUCTIONS An IUCD is usually put in either towards the end of your period or a few days after. It can be fitted up to day 19 in a 28-day menstrual cycle. The doctor or nurse will examine you internally to find the position and size of your womb before they fit an IUCD. They must make sure there is no chance of you being pregnant before they fit an IUCD. Sometimes they will check for any possible existing infection.

There are different types and sizes of IUCD to suit different women. It can be uncomfortable having an IUCD fitted and you might want to have a painkiller or a local anaesthetic.

You may get a period-type pain and some light bleeding for a few days after the IUCD is fitted. Painkillers can help with this.

DIY? No, an IUCD must be inserted by a doctor or nurse.

MOST COMMON COCK-UP Not checking for the thread regularly.

Intrauterine System (IUS)

A small T-shaped plastic device which contains the hormone progestogen that is slowly released into the bloodstream, also known as Mirena.

HOW IT WORKS The mucus from your cervix thickens. This makes it difficult for sperm to move through it and reach an egg and makes the lining of your womb thinner, so it is less likely to accept a fertilised egg.

PROTECTION Immediately, if it is fitted in the first seven days of your menstrual cycle. (If it is fitted at any other time, you will need to use an extra contraceptive method for the first seven days Protection lasts up to five years, although you can have it removed any time.

BABY-PROOFING ABILITIES 99 per cent.

STD-PROTECTION None.

SIDE EFFECTS YOU NEED TO KNOW ABOUT: Headaches, acne and breast tenderness, and slight irregular bleeding between periods for the first three months. After that, side effects disappear, periods usually become much lighter and shorter and period pain is nonexistent. There is a possibility of ovarian cysts (see Chapter Two).

DOES IT RUIN THE MOMENT? No.

HASSLE FACTOR Medium. You need to look for the IUS threads monthly, as it can move or be pushed out by your womb. This is more likely soon after it has been put in and you may not know it has happened. You will also need to have your IUS checked four to six weeks after it is put in, and then once a year.

PLEASURE BAROMETER None.

BAD HABIT PENALTIES Having an IUS fitted might be more uncomfortable if you haven't had children, but you can still use one. You can't use one if you have an untreated STD or PID.

OPERATING INSTRUCTIONS An IUS is put in either towards the end of your period or a few days after. The doctor or nurse must make sure there is no chance of you being pregnant before they fit an IUS. You will be examined internally to find the position and size of your womb before the IUS is fitted. You may get a period-type pain and some bleeding for a few days after the IUS is fitted. Painkillers can help with this.

DIY? No, it must be inserted by a doctor or nurse.

MOST COMMON COCK-UP Forgetting to check the threads.

Natural Family Planning (NFP)

Being aware of your fertile time and avoiding sex on those days.

HOW IT WORKS Observing and recording the following indicators each day of your menstrual cycle: your body temperature when you wake up, cervical secretions (cervical mucus), how long your menstrual cycle lasts.

PROTECTION The fertile time lasts for around eight to nine days of each menstrual cycle.

BABY-PROOFING ABILITIES 98 per cent.

STD-PROTECTION None.

SIDE EFFECTS YOU NEED TO KNOW ABOUT None.

CAN IT RUIN THE MOMENT? Not if you're with a long-term partner and fear of catching an STD is going to be minimal.

HASSLE FACTOR High. It takes three to six cycles to learn effectively. You have to keep daily records. Events such as illness, stress and travel may make fertility indicators harder to interpret. You need to avoid intercourse (or use a barrier method) during the fertile time.

PLEASURE BAROMETER You do not use any chemical agents or physical devices.

BAD HABIT PENALTIES Taking your temperature earlier or later than normal, any illness, such as cold or flu, painkilling drugs (even aspirin) can affect temperature.

OPERATING INSTRUCTIONS You need to take your temperature using a special fertility thermometer or digital thermometer before you get out of bed or have anything to eat or drink. This is known as your basal body temperature (BBT) or waking temperature. The fertile time ends when you have recorded temperatures for three days in a row which are higher than all the previous six days. The difference in temperature will be about 0.2 degrees centigrade. Cervical secretions helps identify the start and end of your fertile days. After your period, you may notice a few days when you feel dry. No cervical secretions will be seen or felt. Then the secretions produced by your cervix change in texture and increase in amount. At first, they feel moist, sticky and white or cloudy. This is the start of the fertile time. The secretions then become clearer, wetter, stretchy and slippery, like raw egg white. This is a sign that you are at your most fertile.

DIY? Yes, but your odds of not getting pregnant increase if you receive instruction before using NFP.

MOST COMMON COCK-UP Not doing it correctly – causing its protection statistics to nosedive.

The Patch

A small oestrogen- and progestogen-spiked strip of material that can be worn anywhere on the buttocks, abdomen, upper torso, front and back (excluding the breasts or upper outer arm).

HOW IT WORKS The hormones are absorbed through the skin and each strip lasts one week, blocking ovulation.

PROTECTION If you start using the patch on the first day of your period, it will be effective immediately (otherwise it takes one week to kick in).

BABY-PROOFING ABILITIES 99 per cent.

STI-PROTECTION None.

SIDE EFFECTS YOU NEED TO KNOW ABOUT Pill-like side effects: nausea, breast tenderness, and spotting. More severe menstrual cramps and breast pain compared to the Pill. The patch may also irritate your skin after a while, making it itch (moving the position once a week can help). Your scratching may tear the patch (experts aren't sure if tears lessen the effectiveness of the patch).

CAN IT RUIN THE MOMENT? Only if it falls off – this happens five per cent of the time (it can be reapplied).

HASSLE FACTOR Low. Stick it on and forget about it for one week.

PLEASURE BAROMETER The edges collect brown stuff – like old plasters – after a while, making it grungy. Also, the patch currently only comes in peach tone, so if your colour is other than peaches and cream, there is no chance it will go unnoticed.

BAD HABIT PENALTIES You shouldn't use it if you

smoke, or have a family history of heart disease or have high blood pressure. The patch is less effective in women who weigh more than 90kg (198lbs). Using St John's Wort can lessen its protection.

OPERATING INSTRUCTIONS You wear the patch on the arm, abdomen or buttock for seven days in a row. Then you exchange it for a new patch, which you wear for another week, and so on. After three weeks (and three patches), the fourth week is patch-free. Each new patch should be applied on the same day of each week. You can bathe and swim without it falling off.

DIY? You need a prescription.

MOST COMMON COCK-UP Using lotion and oils, which make it fall off early.

The Combined Pill (AKA The Pill)

Two synthetic hormones, oestrogen and progestogen, in pill form (there are now over 50 varieties on the market).

HOW IT WORKS Prevents ovaries from releasing eggs and alters cervical mucus to block sperm.

PROTECTION 24/7 protection after you've gone through one Pill packet.

BABY-PROOFING ABILITIES 97 per cent.

STD-PROTECTION None.

SIDE EFFECTS YOU NEED TO KNOW ABOUT Upside: makes periods more regular, decreases menstrual cramping and PMS, reduces risk of endometrial and ovarian cancer. Downside: causes breast tenderness, headaches, possible nausea/depression.

CAN IT RUIN THE MOMENT? No.

HASSLE FACTOR Low. You must remember to take it daily.

PLEASURE BAROMETER Some women report higher libido, some have more vaginal dryness – your call.

BAD HABIT PENALTIES Can't be used by women who smoke or have a family history of high blood pressure or heart problems. Can be unreliable for the rest of the month if missed even once or if you're sick.

OPERATING INSTRUCTIONS There are three different kinds of combined Pills:

Monophasic/21-day Pill. This is the most common. You take one Pill a day for 21 days then no Pills for the next seven days. Each Pill has the same amount of hormone in it.

Phasic Pills. You have two or three sections of different coloured Pills in the pack. They contain different amounts of hormone so you must take them in the right order. You take one Pill a day for 21 days, then no pills for the next seven days.

Every Day Pill. You take one pill a day for 28 days with no break between packets. There are 21 active Pills and seven inactive Pills which don't contain any hormones. You must take these Pills in the right order.

DIY? A prescription is needed.

MOST COMMON COCK-UP Forgetting to take it at the same time, in the correct order or not at all.

The Mini Pill

The synthetic hormone progestogen in pill form.

HOW IT WORKS Alters cervical mucus to block sperm and prevents fertilised eggs from being implanted in the uterus.

PROTECTION Good to go after using one packet, then permanent as long as taking it.

BABY-PROOFING ABILITIES 99 per cent.

STD-PROTECTION None.

SIDE EFFECTS YOU NEED TO KNOW ABOUT May cause spotting between periods, weight gain, breast tenderness.

CAN IT RUIN THE MOMENT? No.

HASSLE FACTOR Low. You must remember to take daily at same time, even when you are menstruating.

PLEASURE BAROMETER None.

BAD HABIT PENALTIES May be less effective in women who weigh over 70kg. Not for the procrastinator.

OPERATING INSTRUCTIONS Swallow at the same time every day.

DIY? You need a prescription.

MOST COMMON COCK-UP Forgetting to take it at the right time. If you're more than three hours late in taking it, you could become pregnant.

Spermicide

Creams, foams, jellies, contraceptive films, foaming vaginal tablets or suppositories which kill sperm before it reaches an egg. Used with diaphragms and cervical caps and can be used with a condom as well.
HOW IT WORKS killer chemicals are released when spermicide is inserted one hour to ten minutes before sex.
PROTECTION One hour after application.
BABY-PROOFING ABILITIES 70 per cent.
STD-PROTECTION None.
SIDE EFFECTS YOU NEED TO KNOW ABOUT It can cause irritation in some people.
CAN IT RUIN THE MOMENT? No.
HASSLE FACTOR High. Messy; also, except for aerosols, you have to wait 10–15 minutes before having sex and they're only good for an hour so if you have sex after that time frame, you've got to do the whole thing again.
PLEASURE BAROMETER Acts as a lubricant.
BAD HABIT PENALTIES None.
OPERATING INSTRUCTIONS For foams, shake container vigorously for at least 20–30 times just before insertion. Take careful aim – you need to have a megadose of spermicide in ready and waiting, EXACTLY in the right place when he spurts or it doesn't work. For jelly, tablets, suppository, film or cream, fill the applicator and lie down to insert it into the vagina until the tip is at or near the cervix; push the applicator plunger to release spermicide. After each use, wash the applicator with soap and water.

Spermicide film should be folded in half and inserted with dry fingers near the cervix, or the film will stick to the fingers and not the cervix.

You can also put a small blob of spermicide gel or cream on his penis right before putting a condom on to boost your protection.

Use more spermicide each time you have sex.
DIY? Yes.
MOST COMMON COCK-UP Having sex too soon after application.

The Sponge

A round polyurethane sponge about 6cm (2^1/$_2$in) in diameter and 2cm (^{3}/$_4$ in) thick, with an indentation in the centre and a small strap to grab or hook your finger around for ease of removal.
HOW IT WORKS The sponge is saturated with a triple-threat sperm-killing gel containing nonoxynol-9, sodium cholate and benzalkonium chloride. It covers the cervix, absorbs the sperm and effectively nukes them.
PROTECTION Immediate and lasts up to 24 hours.
BABY-PROOFING ABILITIES 90 per cent.
STD-PROTECTION None. In fact, nonoxynol-9 has been associated with an increase in some STDs (see Chapter Eight).
SIDE EFFECTS YOU NEED TO KNOW ABOUT Some women get thrush when using the sponge.
CAN IT RUIN THE MOMENT? No, you have at least 24 hours to put it in place.
HASSLE FACTOR Low. It's no-mess, no-fuss and hormone free. It must stay in place at least six hours after sex. However, it can tear or shred inside you and you wouldn't know it.
PLEASURE BAROMETER Unlimited sex per application.
BAD HABIT PENALTIES You might expel it too early during a bowel movement.
OPERATING INSTRUCTIONS It's inserted into the vagina at least 15 minutes and up to 24 hours before sex.
DIY? Yes.
MOST COMMON COCK-UP Leaving it in too long.

Sterilisation

Sterilisation (called vasectomy in men) works by stopping the egg and the sperm meeting.
HOW IT WORKS This is done by blocking the fallopian tubes (which carry an egg from the ovary to the womb) in women or the vas deferens (the tube that carries sperm from the testicles to the penis) in men.
PROTECTION Permanent.

BABY-PROOFING ABILITIES 100 per cent.

STI-PROTECTION None.

SIDE EFFECTS YOU NEED TO KNOW ABOUT
The scrotum may become bruised, swollen and painful. Wearing tight-fitting underpants to support the scrotum day and night for a week will relieve this.

Occasionally, some men have bleeding, a large swelling, or an infection. In this case, see your doctor. Sometimes sperm may leak out of the tube and collect in the surrounding tissue. This may cause inflammation and pain immediately or a few weeks or months later. If this happens it can be treated.

CAN IT RUIN THE MOMENT? No.

HASSLE FACTOR Low. Once you get the operation and are checked to see it has taken, you won't have to worry about contraception ever again.

PLEASURE BAROMETER None.

BAD HABIT PENALTIES Changing your mind. There is an operation to reverse sterilisation, but it is complicated, expensive and may not work.

OPERATING INSTRUCTIONS Male sterilisation is a simple operation and takes about 10–15 minutes. He is given a local anaesthetic. The doctor will make a small cut(s) in the skin of the scrotum, to reach the tubes and will remove a small piece of each tube, or cut the tubes and close the ends. The cuts in the scrotum will be very small and may not need any stitches. After a vasectomy, it usually takes a few months for all the live sperm to disappear from the semen.

For women, there are several ways of blocking the fallopian tubes: tying (ligation); removing a small piece of the tube (excision); sealing (cauterisation); or applying clips or rings.

Laparoscopy is the most common. You will be given a general anaesthetic, or possibly a local anaesthetic. A doctor will make two tiny cuts, one just below your navel and the other just above the bikini line. They will then insert a laparoscope which lets them clearly see your reproductive organs. They will seal or block your fallopian tubes, usually with clips or rings.

For a mini-laparotomy you will usually have to have a general anaesthetic and spend a couple of days in hospital. The doctor will make a small cut in your abdomen, usually just below the bikini line, to reach your fallopian tubes.

To avoid pregnancy you must use contraception right up to the time you are sterilised and until you have your first period after the sterilisation. Your ovaries, womb and cervix are left in place, so you will still release an egg, but it is absorbed by the body.

DIY? No.

MOST COMMON COCK-UP Not going for the follow-up appointments to make sure the operation was a success.

The Vaginal Ring
A clear flexible two-inch ring.

HOW IT WORKS Releases a low-dose oestrogen-progestogen mix of hormones that is absorbed into your system, preventing ovulation (you take it out the week of your period, but you're still protected).

PROTECTION As long as it is inserted.

BABY-PROOFING ABILITIES 99 per cent.

STD-PROTECTION None.

SIDE EFFECTS YOU NEED TO KNOW ABOUT
Headaches, vaginal irritation, discharge, or infection, the ring may accidentally slip out during sex.

CAN IT RUIN THE MOMENT? No. If you or your partner can feel the ring during sex, simply remove it. You can safely go without the device for two hours and not risk protection.

HASSLE FACTOR Low. It's easy to put in but harder to take out because it can be difficult to reach the ring.

PLEASURE BAROMETER It's rounded for comfort, and it also has a hole in the middle so it won't block normal vaginal discharge.

BAD HABIT PENALTIES None. You're even still protected from pregnancy if you vomit (unlike the Pill).

OPERATING INSTRUCTIONS You insert the rubber ring yourself. But because it's not a barrier method, you don't need to place it exactly over the cervix.

DIY? Just need a prescription. It is one-size-fits-all, so it doesn't need to be fitted.

MOST COMMON COCK-UP Forgetting to remove it during your period.

BOOKS

THE CONTRACEPTION SOURCEBOOK
(McGraw-Hill Publishing Co., 2001)
by Elizabeth B. Connell
With more options in contraception than ever before, it's important to know which one will suit you the most. This book will help you do that.

TAKING CHARGE OF YOUR FERTILITY: THE DEFINITIVE GUIDE TO NATURAL BIRTH CONTROL, PREGNANCY ACHIEVEMENT, AND REPRODUCTIVE HEALTH
(Perennial Currents, 2001)
by Tpni Weschler
This comprehensive book explains in lucid, assured terms how to practice the fertility awareness method (FAM), a natural, scientifically proven but little-known form of birth control (which is not to be confused "rhythm" method).

THE PILL AND OTHER FORMS OF HORMONAL CONTRACEPTION: THE FACTS
(OUP, 1997)
by John Guillebaud.
Classic and regularly-updated handbook by the UK's leading expert on oral contraception.

CONTRACEPTION: A USER'S HANDBOOK
(OUP, 1997)
By Anne Szarewski and John Guillebaud
Your choices, plus an explanation of their availability, ease of use and effectiveness.

ABORTION: WHOSE RIGHT?
(Hodder Arnold, 2002)
Edited by Ellie Lee .
Looks at the situation in the UK since the 1997 Abortion Act.

FERTILITY AND CONCEPTION: THE COMPLETE GUIDE TO GETTING PREGNANT
(Dorling Kindersley, 2003)
by Zita West
Comprehensive and user friendly, with a guide to fertility treatments.

INFORMATION AND ADVICE

Marie Stopes International (MSI)
www.mariestopes.org.uk
Your round-the-world site (currently has an
address in 30 countries) for info on
contraceptives.

Condomania
www.condomania.com
Carries every condom made under the sun and
will not only tell you how to use them – they'll
send them to you wherever you are.

SafeSense
www.condoms.net
Offers a full array of products from the best, most
recognised manufacturers as well as tips and
ideas for choosing and using.

The Family Planning Association
www.fpa.org.uk/guide/contracep/condom.htm
Immediate info on your contraceptive choices in
the UK.

The Emergency Contraception Website
www.NOT-2-LATE.com
Provides accurate information about emergency
contraception derived in several languages.

Planned Parenthood Federation of America
(PPFA)
www.plannedparenthood.org
The world's largest reproductive healthcare
organisation.

The Brook Centres
www.brook.org.uk/
A network of advice centres in the UK on
contraception and unplanned pregnancy, primarily
aimed at younger women.

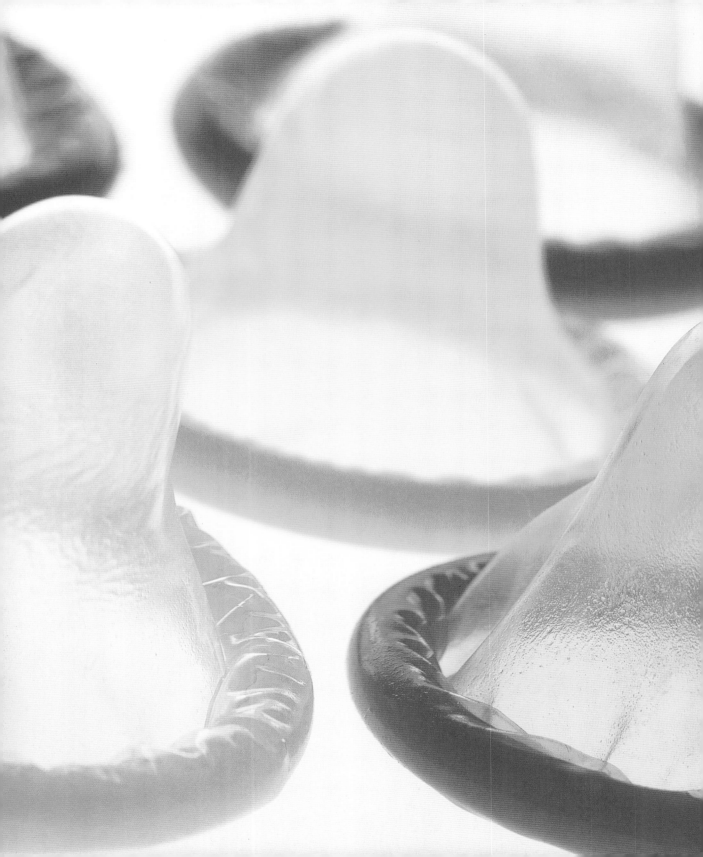

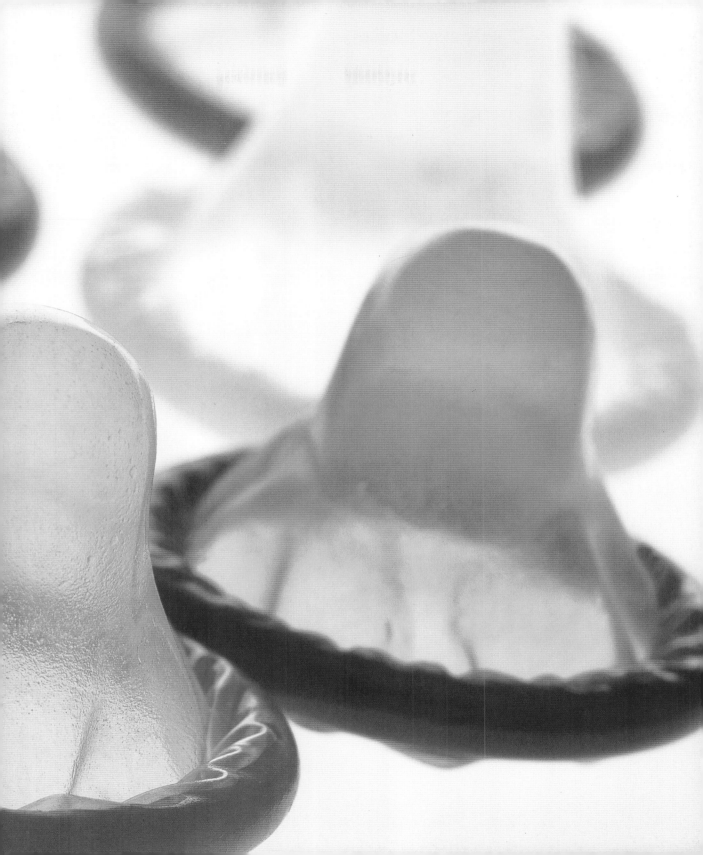

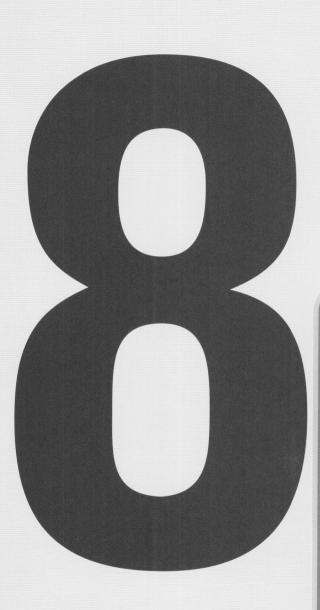

5 Healthy STD-Prevention Habits

(**1**) Get tested. If you have any STD risk at all, make sure you include a screening in your annual gynaecological check-up.

(**2**) Remember, you're not just having sex with that person… but with everyone they've slept with, and everyone they've slept with…

(**3**) Don't rely on finding symptoms. Many of the most common STDs, especially HPV, chlamydia, and herpes, produce no obvious symptoms in up to 75 per cent of those infected. You're much more likely to notice if you've contracted trichomoniasis, thrush, or bacterial vaginosis (which causes an unusual discharge), gonorrhoea (which makes it painful to urinate), or syphilis (which is signalled by a tell-tale sore).

(**4**) Don't have sex with someone new when drunk. You are less likely to use a condom or use one correctly.

(**5**) Know when to use what.

SEX PLAGUES

Everything you need to know about sexually transmitted diseases.

Have you ever had a sexually transmitted infection? Not you, no way. But odds are that you have. There are 12 million new cases of STDs every year, globally. If you or your lover have just four other sexual partners in your lifetime, you will almost definitely be one of those infected. So even if you think it's impossible that the person you are getting naked with has an STD – the stats aren't exactly in your favour. Nor will condoms always keep you safe. Though they're still essential for preventing STDs like HIV and gonorrhoea, they won't necessarily protect you from genital herpes or warts.

  Wake-up call: there are more than 20 kinds of STDs and they are transmitted in different ways. While sexual intercourse is the highest risk activity for all types of STDs – herpes and hepatitis, for example, can be passed through kissing. That is why no form of getting to know someone physically is entirely risk free – from smooching to foreplay to oral, anal, or vaginal intercourse.

KEEP YOUR PANTS ON

Why are women more likely to be infected than men?

Part of the reason for this unfair state of things is that a woman comes into contact with more fluid from ejaculation than a man does from vaginal secretions. If the ejaculate is infected with an STD, a woman gets that much more exposure. Also, diseases like gonorrhoea, chlamydia and trichomoniasis (and possibly AIDS) infect the body through specific disease-friendly 'target tissue'. During sex, a lot less of this type of tissue is exposed in a man (it lines his urethra but only if the tip of the urethra is exposed) than in a woman (it lines her entire vagina and covers her cervix). For unknown reasons, menstruation also seems to be a factor. The risk of infection by HIV and of PID caused by gonorrhoea increases during your time of the month.

How can I protect myself against an STD with a new partner?

In terms of risk, you are, in effect, sleeping not only with this man but with all of his current and former partners, so he could indirectly expose you to infections from many people.

Which is why the only real safe way to proceed is simply to assume that a potential partner is infected until you know for sure that he isn't. Awkward as it may be, you have to find a way to talk about STDs and sex and you have to do it before things get hot and heavy. Failure to do so may have some serious consequences: one study found that women who never raised the STD subject before they had sex were three times more likely to have an infection than those who did.

Once you do decide to have sex, always use a latex or polyurethane condom, correctly, every time. For vaginal sex, anal sex and oral sex. Even if you're using another form of birth control for pregnancy prevention (STD prevention and pregnancy protection are two separate issues).

I make sure the guys I sleep with wear condoms, so why should I worry?

Condoms are effective in preventing diseases that are spread by blood and body fluids – gonorrhoea, chlamydia, HIV and hepatitis B, for example. They don't work as well for viruses spread by skin-to-skin contact, like herpes, genital warts and syphilis if the infection is hanging out in areas that a condom does not cover – at the base of and around the genitals. And when an STD is spread through kissing, a condom is useless.

Do I have to tell someone I have an STD?

Wouldn't you want to know? The good news is that most bugs are completely curable or avoidable. Make sure you drop your bomb before sex – and before you're naked. You don't need to go into details. The important thing is to tell him what level your STD is at and explain how you're going to make sure that he isn't at risk.

Oral sex is safe, right?

Wake up, Sleeping Beauty. Oral sex is a relatively low-risk activity, but it isn't exactly safe sex. People carry all sorts of viruses and bacteria in their mouths. Among the most common diseases transmitted during oral sex:

- Thrush: Up to one third of all of all adults are thought to harbour the fungus that causes thrush in their mouths, which may explain why women who receive a tongue lashing twice a week or more have triple the risk of getting thrush (see Chapter Two).
- HSV: There are two main of HSV and both can cause oral and genital herpes.
- Hepatitis B: If you haven't been vaccinated.
- Chlamydia: If your partner has this bacteria in his

> Your risk of disease from one bout of unprotected sex: about 33% – that's one in three. Think about it. Here's how it breaks down, from most likely to least: herpes, genital warts, chlamydia, gonorrhoea, HIV, Hepatitis B, and syphilis.

ARE YOU STD SAVVY?

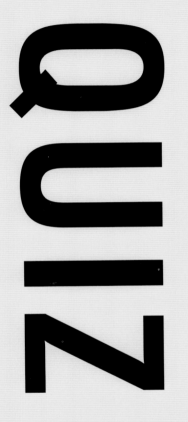

QUESTIONS

① **Which of the following condoms help provide protection against pregnancy and most STD's:**
a Condoms lubricated with spermicide
b Condoms marked 'Sensitive'
c Condoms marked 'Extra Strength'
d Condoms for women (aka female condom)
e All of the above

② **Which of the following STDs can be cured?**
a Chlamydia
b Herpes
c HPV
d HIV
e Hepatitis B

③ **If you forgot to use a condom and begin to feel a burning sensation in your genitals, you could possibly be infected with which of the following:**
a Herpes
b HPV
c Gonorrhoea
d Chlamydia

④ **Which of the following STDs cannot be passed on through oral sex?**
a Herpes
b Genital warts
c HIV/AIDS
d Chlamydia
e Pubic lice
f Gonorrhoea

⑤ **There is a single test which screens for all the STIs at once.** True or False?

ANSWERS

1 (e) The only condoms that don't give protection are those made of lambskin or novelty condoms (such as flavoured or coloured ones) that don't have any protection. guarantees on their packaging

2 (a) Chlamydia – all of the other infections are viruses which can be treated but not cured.

3 Trick question – it could be any STD, even one not listed.

4 (e) Pubic lice – which is why it's important to use a dental dam for oral sex.

5 False: in fact, every STD has a specific and different test. Some infections get detected with a swab of cells, others through urine tests, others with a visual exam, and still others (such as HIV) with a blood test.

SAFE SEX

Safe sex kit

- Five condoms, preferably not spermicidal, and in a variety of the styles you like.
- One bottle of latex-safe, water-based lubricant (available in both single-use tubes and a variety of flavours).
- Five pairs of latex (or latex-alternative) gloves
- Five dental dams or a box of clingfilm.
- A tube of aloe vera gel (helps soothe skin irritated from latex or lubricants).

Are you at risk

- Were you born a woman?
- Were there twenty or less birthday candles on your last cake?
- Is your town big enough that you don't know everyone who lives there?
- Did you get down and dirty with more than one man in the past three months?
- Did you get lucky with someone new in the last three months?
- Are you still waiting to have the safe sex talk with your lover?
- Is he a sleep-around sort of hound-dog?
- Do you sometimes skip suiting him up?
- Have you ever had an STD?
- Have you ever had a one-night stand?
- Have you ever been wasted and had sex?
- Have you ever done it up the bum?

The more 'yes' answers, the higher your risk of getting an STD.

throat, there is a small chance you could contract it through his saliva during oral sex.
- Syphilis: The risk of contracting syphilis is high during the early stages of infection, when lesions are most active. After about a year three, transmission is less likely.
- HIV: If your partner has HIV-positive blood in his mouth and you have cuts in your vagina, there is a remote chance he could infect you. Your risk increases if he ejaculates when you go south on him.

The best protection is to cover up before you start snacking. If you're on the giving end, slip a condom on him first. You can use a flavoured one (but check to make sure it specifically states that it protects against STDs – some taster's choices are novelty items and don't offer these guarantees).

> You can get an STD from sharing towels or sex toys.

While your being on the receiving end is less risky for both of you, you can up your protection by using a dental dam – flat pieces of latex about the size of a slice of bread. But they're hard to keep in place and saliva and vaginal secretions can leak around the edges. Making a DIY-dam (by cutting the tip off a condom and slitting it up the middle, then flattening it over your opening) doesn't work any better. However, wrapping your vagina in clingfilm is fairly effective.

SCRATCH 'N' SNIFF

I can't seem to stop scratching my vagina. Is it thrush or an STD?

You can't tell. This is why it isn't really a good idea to use over-the-counter thrush medications (see Chapter Two). You may end up missing a more serious infection which could result in PID and possibly infertility.

Can You Tell If A Man Has An STD Just By Looking At Him?

Get real! Unless he has a 'Beware! Toxic Site' sign hanging off his penis, there is no failsafe way to make sure he is in the clear. But taking a good look at his privates may give you a clue:

IF YOU NOTICE	IT COULD BE	PROTECT YOURSELF	GET A CLEAN BILL OF HEALTH
Flesh-coloured bumps	Genital warts	Wait until he's had them removed and been given the all-clear by his doctor before having sex.	Get a check-up. There are over 120 strains of HPV.
A mild red or flesh-coloured rash	Syphilis or HIV	Some rashes are harmless, but the symptoms of syphilis along with swollen lymph glands and feet could signal a recent HIV infection.	Get tested and get tested again in three months.
Something moving	Crabs	Avoid any skin-to-skin contact until everything is decontaminated.	Look for any unusual movement in your vaginal area.
A yellow, green or watery discharge	Gonorrhoea, chlamydia or trichomoniasis	If you've touched the discharge, wash your hands immediately to prevent infecting other areas.	Get any unusual vaginal discharge checked out.
Teeny blister-like sores.	Herpes Simplex Virus (HSV).	Avoid having sex during his outbreak.	Get tested. Herpes can be transmitted by skin-to-skin contact even when blisters aren't visible.

Call Your Doctor Now Checklist

...if you have any of the following symptoms:

1. Abnormal or smelly discharges from the vagina, penis, rectum.
2. Unexplained genital bleeding.
3. Pain when you pee or have sex.
4. Genital itching.
5. Noticeable bumps, rashes, swelling or blisters anywhere in the genital area.

I keep on getting BV (bacterial vaginosis) even though I take my full course of antibiotics.

You're in the unlucky 50 per cent group for whom antibiotics don't work when it comes to curing BV. You've got a few choices:

- Try a different type of antibiotic.
- Try acetic acid vaginal jelly (Aci-Jel). It may inhibit the excessive growth of Gardnerella and Mobiluncus and help restore your vagina's natural balance of bacteria by restoring its acidity. Available without a prescription from most chemists, the pack contains a special applicator for inserting the jelly into the vagina – use one applicatorful, twice a day. Unfortunately, it isn't known if Aci-Jel damages condoms and contraceptive diaphragms or caps.

Orally transmitted gonorrhoea is on the rise in the UK

- Try live yogurt (it says 'live' on the pot). This contains live friendly lactobacilli bacteria, which are reduced in numbers in BV. Gently smear a small amount of yogurt over the vulva (the area around the opening of the vagina), and also put some inside the vagina by pushing a tampon

THE SILENT TYPES

While you may already know that you need to 'fess up if you have any of the H-triplets: HIV, HPV (genital warts) and HSV, other infections are not such obvious tell-alls:

Trichomoniasis
- If you do get infected, make sure he gets checked out as well and use a condom until you've finished the course of antibiotics or else the infection will just bounce back and forth between you.

Thrush
- While it's pretty unlikely you'll give it to him, the yeast toxins can make his penis burn or break out in a rash. Also, condoms are a no-go since the thrush medication can erode the latex, even if it's been applied a few days before you have sex.

Four steps to damming up your vagina:
- Give the dam a rinse to wash away the powder covering it, otherwise he may get dry mouth and you an irritation.
- Mark the up side with a permanent marker. This way you won't end up mixing up the side that's been touching your vaginal lips with the one his lips have been touching if the damn thing drops as you buck with pleasure.
- Add a spot of lube to your vagina to keep things juicy.
- Lay it down, making sure it covers the entire area (dams can be on the lightweight size). Hold it in place to prevent it from slipping.

back inside its applicator and adding about a teaspoonful of yogurt in the space. Then insert the tampon in the usual way, which will push the yogurt into the top of the vagina. Remove the tampon an hour later. Do this twice a day for a week.

> BV doubles the likelihood of a premature birth.

PERMANENT VISITORS

I have been with my boyfriend for two years he swears he's never cheated. So how come I recently got diagnosed with genital warts? Should I be looking for a new boyfriend?

Hold off. Either you or your boyfriend could have had an earlier case of 'microscopic warts' (visible only with the use of special instruments) which disappeared for awhile (common with genital warts) and recently resurfaced.

My new boyfriend just told me that he had genital warts more than four years ago. He says he's safe because nothing has happened since. Should I be wary?

Chances are you're safe. Though genital warts are extremely common and highly contagious, most people's immune systems are capable of completely wiping them out. The longer he's gone without a wart, the more likely it is that he is in the clear.

But because there are so many different types of HPV, no test can conclusively tell you that your partner or you are HPV-free. And in as many as 90 per cent of cases, genital warts cause no noticeable symptoms. So even though it won't protect you 100 per cent, you should still use a condom.

This guy I met told me he has herpes. Will I get it if I have sex with him?

Yes, unless you play smart. Herpes, like genital warts, can't be cured. But, again like genital warts, it can be controlled – and, therefore, avoided by new playmates. A person with herpes should take antiviral medication, which lessens the symptoms and controls or even prevent outbreaks. To avoid getting it from your new lover, don't have sex if he has an outbreak or visible sores. Wait till they clear. Once they do, you're cleared for take-off, but make sure he or you wear a condom. The virus can be passed to you whether it is inactive or not.

Can I give my boyfriend genital herpes when I have a cold sore on my mouth?

Stay north of the waistline if there's a cold sore in the vicinity. Cold sores or fever blisters are the infection, formerly known as oral herpes, caused by a Herpes Simplex Virus-1 (HSV-1) infection. Genital herpes is mainly caused by HSV-2. Nearly a third of genital herpes cases are in fact caused by HSV-1, almost always transmitted via oral-genital contact, from the person with the infected mouth.

So avoid all skin contact when a sore is present. It's also possible to spread the virus even without sores. For about two-to-five days each year, your body goes through what's called viral shedding, in which it releases a small amount of virus through the skin wherever it is infected. During this time, the virus still travels along the nerves to skin and mucous membrane sites. Because your body gives you no

> Itching in the genital area can be a sign of gonorrhoea, syphilis, trichomoniasis, BV and herpes. Discharge also signals chlamydia.

warning, such as minor pain, discomfort, or a tingling sensation in the skin where the shedding is going on, there's no way of knowing when it is taking place. You usually get four or five herpes attacks per year; gradually, they will lessen in severity, and the intervals between them will grow longer.

I had unprotected sex over a year ago and I've never had any symptoms, so what are the chances I have an STD?

You don't need to be sick to get sick. Some common STDs do their dirty work in women without causing any noticeable problems.

Take genital warts: three weeks after exposure to the virus, which can be passed by any skin-to-skin contact (not only through sex), some women develop genital warts. But most have no idea they're infected. Only a small number will find out months or even years down the road, when their doctors report they have an abnormal cervical smear. And while only a few HPV strains have the potential to cause the abnormal cell growth linked with cancer, those strains can be deadly. If left untreated, these dangerous strains can cause mutations in cervical (and occasionally vaginal) cells that in some cases can lead to cancer.

As for chlamydia, although roughly one in 11 sexually active young women is currently infected with this quiet virus, and most have absolutely no symptoms. Even the 20 per cent who are likely to experience abdominal pain, slight discharge or bleeding after sex within one to three weeks of contracting chlamydia don't necessarily make the link between cramping and having an STD. Which is why you should get tested for chlamydia at least once a year and whenever you start having sex with a new partner. The disease is easily treatable with antibiotics.

> Stress, illness, menstruation, pregnancy, temperature extremes, exhaustion, temperature changes, sunbathing, and sexual intercourse can all trigger a herpes attack.

In most women who have it, chlamydia travels no further than the cervix. But in about one in ten, it travels further upwards through the uterus (womb) into the Fallopian tubes, where it can cause an inflammation known as PID – which may be painful but can occur without any pain at all. If the infection istreated at this stage, the tube may recover. But one

WHEN IT GETS SERIOUS

Genital Warts and Cancer
Even though they cause 93 per cent of cervical cancer cases, genital warts don't always spell cancer. Generally, 30 per cent of women with genital warts develop lesions and only 10 per cent of women with lesions develop cervical cancer.

Herpes Complex
Other places you can get herpes:

- Herpes simplex keratitis is an infection of the eye that is caused by touching it after coming into contact with a herpes sore. Repeated infections can scar the eye and affect your vision. Topical antiviral medications are usually prescribed for treatment.
- Herpetic whitlow, a painful infection of the fingertip, is caused by touching herpes sores. Antiviral medications are given to prevent transmission.
- The herpes virus that causes chicken pox can lead to shingles. After you have had chicken pox as a child, the virus can lie dormant in nerve cells near your spinal cord or brain. Ageing, illness, or stress can reactivate the virus causing a band of blisters your body that heals within a month. Antiviral medications can help prevent serious complications.

in five women who have PID through an STD eventually becomes infertile, often due to the scarring that the chronic infection causes. And since it's the scarring that causes the problems even after treatment with antibiotics, many women never regain their fertility. The more times you have PID, the more likely you will end up infertile or suffering an ectopic pregnancy.

Another silent but deadly STD is hepatitis B. You may not think of hepatitis B as a sexually transmitted infection, but it's 100 times more contagious than HIV, and about one in every 20 people will be infected at some point in their life. In most adults, the immune system springs into action at the first contact with the virus, killing it before it does any serious damage to the liver, and spurring the body to manufacture antibodies to ward off the disease in the future. But in up to 10 per cent of the people infected, the disease takes hold.

Those people, called chronic carriers, have the disease for life and are more prone to cirrhosis, a life-threatening disease that scars the liver. They also have a 200-times greater chance of liver cancer than people without the disease.

> A nipple that suddenly becomes inverted can be a sign of a cancer underneath it, so you should see your doctor straight away.

Gonorrhoea also sneaks up on women. Although easily curable with one-dose antibiotics, untreated it can cause PID, ectopic pregnancy and increased risk of HIV infection.

Bringing us to the last on the list of silent STDs. HIV may take as long as ten years to develop into AIDS. During that time, you may have no signs of illness or you may experience fatigue and flu-like symptoms. AIDS is controllable, but not curable and will eventually lead to death.

I had chlamydia and got treatment, but now I am always in pain.

Chlamydia, PID, gonorrhoea and genital warts can trigger persistent pelvic pain in about 30 per cent of women, even after they have received treatment. Here are some of the reasons it happens and what you should do to avoid it:

- Get routinely screened for STDs: Because so many STDs flourish without obvious symptoms, they can cause scarring that can be painful, affect your fertility and increase your risk of ectopic pregnancy Also, you may have two or more STDs but have

been diagnosed and treated for only one.

- If you have a bacterial STD, have a follow-up after treatment to make sure the medication worked: Some STDs – like gonorrhoea – have become resistant to common antibiotics.
- Ask your lover to get checked: STDs – especially chlamydia – can have a ping-pong effect, bouncing between partners before one or the other

> The breast extends from the armpit, called the axilla by doctors, down to the sixth rib bone.

COULD YOU HAVE AN STD AND NOT KNOW IT?

Some symptoms of STDs are eerily like those of other kinds of infections. They may not even show up in the genital area. Here is your See Your Doctor Now checklist:

- Weight loss that is constant, rapid, or unexplained
- Abdominal pain
- Appetite loss
- Chills
- Diarrhoea
- Aching joints
- Bowel problems
- Vomiting
- Fatigue
- Fevers
- Headaches
- Night sweats
- Muscular pain
- Swollen glands
- Sore throat complications.

is completely cured. You are more likely to suffer pelvic pain if you are infected a second or third time.

THE KILLERS

I'm dating someone who is HIV positive. How high are my chances of contracting it if we are careful?

There are no 100 per cent guarantees but one study showed that among couples where one of the duet is HIV-positive, none of the HIV-free partners were infected when they always – and correctly (see Chapter Seven) used condoms. One in ten of the HIV-negative partners became infected among those who were not so religious about suiting up.

There are 36.1 million cases of AIDS around the world.

My boyfriend claims he is HIV-negative because his blood donations have never been rejected. Is that a safe assumption?

It depends on a couple of things. Firstly, how regularly he donates blood – the longer the gap between donations, the less he can rely on this method of deciding his HIV status. And secondly, when was the last time he donated blood – test results may not reliably show up as positive for at least several weeks to several months after exposure.

I've heard that as my number of sexual partners increases, so does my risk of getting cervical cancer. Why?

While you can't 'catch' cancer, you can put yourself more at risk for it. The more sexual partners you have, the greater your risk of getting STDs, which up your risk of getting cervical cancer. Chlamydia, for example, puts women up to 6.6 times more at risk for developing cervical cancer; and women with genital warts are ten times more likely to develop it. Since many STDs are asymptomatic, you could be on your way to cervical cancer and other reproductive problems without even knowing it. Your best defence is to get a yearly gynaecological exam, cervical smear and STD testing.

It is estimated that 41,200 people are living with HIV in the United Kingdom, around a third of whom are undiagnosed.

THE LOW-DOWN

Left untreated, STDs can cause lasting damage, including infertility; some, such as HIV, can even be fatal. Your best defence? Aside from celibacy, it's having the knowledge you need.

AIDS

THE DOWN-LOW The end product of becoming infected with HIV (Human Immunodeficiency Virus) – a virus that attacks your body's immune system by infecting your white blood cells (the protecting ones), eventually crippling your ability to fight off illness.

TRANSLATION You can carry HIV and not have signs of AIDS, although you'll probably develop it. Every 60 seconds, five people under age 24 become infected.

TRANSMISSION COMPLETE Through body fluids (blood, saliva, semen or vaginal secretions or breast milk), through anal and vaginal intercourse or oral sex, shared needles used for injecting IV drugs or accidental pricks with infected needles, blood transfusions, childbirth or breastfeeding.

ETA AIDS can take from six months to ten years to develop. You'll test HIV-positive during this time, but may have no symptoms.

YOU'VE GOT IT You might have no symptoms for years or, shortly after infection, you may experience a flu-like illness, followed by a period of feeling good (but you're still contagious). Other early signs include extreme fatigue, fever, weight loss, diarrhoea, night sweats. The only way to know for sure is through a blood test to screen for antibodies.

TO GET RID OF IT You can't. But early detection with a blood test and new drugs may prolong life.

PENALTY Death.

TAKE ACTION Using a condom during any type of intercourse and/or blowjobs, and a dental dam if he goes down on you.

WEIRD FACT Because it can take up to three months or more for the antibodies to appear, a negative test should always be repeated.

Bacterial Vaginosis (BV)

THE DOWN-LOW An imbalance, including pH changes, in the vagina when different types of bacteria outnumber the normal and healthy bacteria. The cause of this disruption in the balance of the vaginal flora is not fully understood, as BV is not always sexually transmitted.

TRANSLATION You may not get it from having sex but women who are sexually active are more likely to get BV, especially if they have more than one sleeping partner or have switched men lately.

TRANSMISSION COMPLETE Any time you introduce different bacteria to the vaginal environment, usually through unprotected vaginal or anal intercourse, unprotected manual sex, or double dipping a condom for vaginal intercourse and anal intercourse.

YOU'VE GOT IT You might not know. Half of women who have it have no symptoms. The other half have excessive fishy-smelling (especially after sex) heavy, creamy greyish-white vaginal discharge plus itchiness and possible swelling, and there may be a bit of redness.

TO GET RID OF IT Antibiotics.

PENALTY Once you get it, you're more likely to get it again. It puts you at risk for other infections.

TAKE ACTION Practice proper hygiene, sexually and otherwise, and limit your number of partners.

WEIRD FACT Douching and/or wiping badly after a bowel movement may increase the risk.

Chlamydia

THE DOWN-LOW A bacterial infection which infects the cervix and can spread to the urethra, Fallopian tubes, and ovaries in women.

TRANSLATION One of the fastest-spreading STDs out there.

TRANSMISSION COMPLETE Having vaginal, anal or oral sex without a condom.

ETA One to three weeks for symptoms to show up, if at all.

YOU'VE GOT IT A milky yellow vaginal discharge, genital itching/burning, dull stomach pain, and pain during peeing. But up to 75 per cent of those infected have no symptoms at all.

TO GET RID OF IT A five-day course of antibiotics cures it. But both you AND your partner need treatment before resuming sex. Otherwise, it'll just leapfrog back and forth between you.

PENALTY Infertility, abnormal cervical smears, PID or cervical infections.

TAKE ACTION Only condoms offer protection, but even they aren't 100 per cent effective.

WEIRD FACT Men are just as likely to be infected as women. Chlamydia is often misdiagnosed as gonorrhoea, so many people take the wrong antibiotic.

Genital Warts

THE DOWN-LOW There are more than 100 different known strains of human papillomavirus (HPV), a viral infection of the genital area or rectum.

TRANSLATION Bumps down there.

TRANSMISSION COMPLETE Unprotected vaginal, oral or anal sex or touching a partner's infected area.

ETA Three weeks to eight months after contact.

YOU'VE GOT IT It shows up as highly contagious, painless smooth and/or cauliflower-like warts around the genitals and anus.

TO GET RID OF IT There's no cure for the infection, but warts can be destroyed with creaming (prescriptive), freezing, burning, lasering or cutting. Warts come back in about 25 per cent of all cases. Regular examinations with cervical smears are your best bet for detection.

PENALTY Certain types of HPV can lead to cervical, penile, anal, and rectal cancers.

TAKE ACTION Genital warts are spread through skin-to-skin contact, so wearing a condom will only protect his penis and (if it's a female condom) your vagina.

WEIRD FACT Warts don't have to be present for HPV to be transmitted.

Gonorrhea – 'The Clap'

THE DOWN-LOW A bacterial infection caused by Neisseria gonorrhoea.

TRANSLATION A bacterial infection.

TRANSMISSION COMPLETE Having unprotected vaginal, oral or anal sex.

ETA If symptoms appear, they appear in women within ten days and from one to 14 days in men.

YOU'VE GOT IT Eighty per cent of women and 10 per cent of men with gonorrhoea show no symptoms. If symptoms do show up, they're usually in the form of a painful burning sensation during peeing and greenish vaginal discharge.

TO GET RID OF IT A short antibiotic course will cure gonorrhoea, but BOTH partners must be treated, even if one doesn't have symptoms. You must also avoid all sexual contact until you're cured.

PENALTY Infertility, arthritis, heart problems, and PID. It's also easier for HIV to infect people with gonorrhoea.

TAKE ACTION Condoms, although diaphragms and cervical caps used with spermicide are also effective.

WEIRD FACT Gonorrhoea can occur in the throat from oral sex as well as in the anus from anal sex, or the eye from not washing your hands after anal sex.

Hepatisis B

THE DOWN-LOW One of an alphabet series of hepatitis viruses (it runs from A on) that cause inflammation of the liver.

TRANSLATION A liver disease.

TRANSMISSION COMPLETE Unprotected sex, sharing drug needles, and getting a tattoo or piercing with dirty tools.

YOU'VE GOT IT Many people have no symptoms or confuse their symptoms with flu: they get a low fever, muscle aches, fatigue, loss of appetite, vomiting and diarrhoea. Later, your urine may be very dark, your bowel movements pale and your eyes and skin will get a yellowish (jaundice) tint.

TO GET RID OF IT Over time, about 90 per cent of people will fight HBV with antibodies and cure themselves. The other 10 per cent never develop antibodies. There's no cure for them, but drugs such as alpha interferon-2B can lessen the symptoms.

PENALTY Cirrhosis of the liver, cancer of the liver.

TAKE ACTION Condoms (though not 100 per cent

effective because hepatitis can be present outside the areas covered by condoms).

WEIRD FACT It's the only STD for which there is a vaccine (Hepatitis B is at least 100 times more infectious than HIV, so the vaccine is worth getting).

Herpes

THE DOWN-LOW There are loads of different types, but the two main strains of the herpes virus you're mostly concerned with are: HSV-1, which generally causes sores in the mouth area, and HSV-2, which mainly causes sores in the genital area. But HSV-1 can also appear genitally and HSV-2 can equally appear in the mouth and face region.

TRANSLATION Herpes and cold sores can be the same virus, so you can get herpes from oral sex with someone with cold sores (or get cold sores from someone with herpes).

TRANSMISSION COMPLETE Rubbing and touching the infected area. The first attack is often the most contagious and painful.

ETA The infection can remain dormant for months, years, even life. But if symptoms do occur, they generally show within one to three weeks of infection, lasting an equal amount of time.

YOU'VE GOT IT Two-thirds of people with HSV-2 don't know they have it. The symptoms are itching, followed by painful blisters that rupture and become tender sores which may make peeing painful. But you can get infected without any symptoms at all, only to have them suddenly pop up years later. Seventy-five per cent of people will also have recurring symptoms, lasting three days to two weeks each time. Often subsequent outbursts are less severe than the initial one.

TO GET RID OF IT No known cure. It can be controlled to a certain extent with prescribed antiviral drugs which may make the sores come back less often and shorten the time they're around when they do return, so they last only a few days.

PENALTY Although a hassle, the worst danger is severe discomfort.

TAKE ACTION Initially, a condom's your best protection against infection. But if you do get herpes, avoid all sexual contact during an outbreak. Don't share towels (or cutlery if you have mouth sores). And if you've ever had a genital herpes infection, use condoms – even when you can't see sores (you're infectious a few days before they appear). Also, if you feel discomfort in the area where the sores appear, use a condom as the pain may mean an outbreak is about to appear. And keep using condoms during an attack until the sores are crusted over.

WEIRD FACT If symptoms do appear, they may fade without treatment, but the sores will unpredictably recur, often when you're under stress or have your period.

Pelvic Inflammatory Disease – PID

THE DOWN-LOW Shorthand for any serious bacterial infection of the reproductive organs that are housed in the pelvis: the uterus, uterine lining, Fallopian tubes, and/or ovaries. These infections usually start in the vagina and, when left untreated, can progressively infect other reproductive organs.

TRANSLATION You can get very sick.

TRANSMISSION COMPLETE PID occurs when a woman has an STD such as chlamydia or gonorrhoea which goes untreated.

ETA A couple of days.

YOU'VE GOT IT There usually aren't any symptoms, or the symptoms are seemingly un-STD related, so they get missed: cramps, tenderness, fever, chills, painful periods that may last longer than previous cycles, unusual vaginal discharge, pain during vaginal intercourse are some of the more common ones.

TO GET RID OF IT Usually strong antibiotics. And lots of them.

PENALTY PID can lead to permanent infertility or ectopic pregnancy and possibly death.

TAKE ACTION Using condoms during vaginal intercourse and getting screened annually for STDs.

WEIRD FACT PID can re-occur even once treated if the person becomes reinfected.

Pubic Lice ('Cabs') and Scabies

THE DOWN-LOW Minute blood-sucking insects that gorge themselves on your blood.

TRANSLATION Little bugs crawling all over your pubic hair and biting you.

TRANSMISSION COMPLETE Pubic lice and scabies are usually — but not always — transmitted by close physical or sexual contact with an infected person. But you can also get them from sharing towels or bedding used by an infected person.

ETA The critters hatch seven to nine days after infection although you may not notice the itching for a few weeks.

YOU'VE GOT IT For pubic lice, tiny white balls around your pubic area, underarms, head, eyebrows and even lashes — basically any place you have body hair. These are the eggs which hatch into the lice, pin-head-sized, greyish-white clawed creatures (unless they've just finished a meal, then they're a dark red colour).

For scabies, severe itching, especially at night. Small red bumps like pimples or lines like small scratches appear where the mite has burrowed into the skin to lay eggs.

TO GET RID OF IT A special shampoo you and your partner lather into your pubic area. You'll also need to sterilise sheets, towels, toilet seats, against re-infection.

PENALTY Your genitals will continue itching and you may experience rashes.

TAKE ACTION Dry-clean materials such as bedding, towels and clothing which you think may carry scabies or pubic lice.

WEIRD FACT Pubic lice are not the same as body lice.

Syphilis

THE DOWN-LOW A bacterial infection of the genitals.

TRANSLATION Red sores on the mouth, penis, vagina, bottom hole, or skin.

TRANSMISSION COMPLETE When someone touches a sore on a person who has syphilis during oral, vaginal, or anal sexual contact.

ETA Three weeks to eight months after infection.

YOU'VE GOT IT There are three stages: Stage one is a painless red sore at the place where your body came into contact with the bacteria. Stage two is headaches, a rash or a fever. Stage three has no symptoms.

TO GET RID OF IT A single dose of penicillin can cure a person who has had syphilis for less than one year. Otherwise longer treatment is necessary. All sexual partners should also be treated.

PENALTY The syphilis organism, 'spirochete', can remain in the body for life and lead to disfigurement, permanent heart/brain/nerve/bone damage, mental illness, and even death. It is also easier for HIV to infect a person who has a syphilis sore.

TAKE ACTION Condoms (though not 100 per cent effective because syphilis can be present outside the areas covered by condoms).

WEIRD FACT There are some really horrid pictures of people with entire arms and legs eaten away by syphilis.

Trichomoniasis — Trich

THE DOWN-LOW Trichomoniasis is a microscopic parasite found all over the world.

TRANSLATION An infection of the vagina caused by a freeloader.

TRANSMISSION COMPLETE Having unprotected vaginal sex.

ETA Four to 20 days after exposure.

YOU'VE GOT IT Almost half of those infected don't have any symptoms. Some women may notice a green-yellowish frothy vaginal discharge and itching.

TO GET RID OF IT Antibiotics for both you and your partner.

PENALTY Because it causes major irritation to your vaginal walls, it can significantly increase your chances of catching HIV.

TAKE ACTION Condoms (though not 100 per cent effective).

WEIRD FACT Natural fluids in the prostate fight the trichomonad parasite, so in some cases trich goes away on its own in men.

5 Questions That Can Be Answered In One Word

① How can you be 100 per cent guaranteed safe from STDs?

Abstinence

② What's the next best defence against STDs?

Condoms

③ If you catch one STD, are you more likely to catch another?

Yes

④ Can washing with soap after sex keep you from catching an STD?

Possibly

⑤ What about douching?

No

BOOKS

SEXUALLY TRANSMITTED DISEASES: A PHYSICIAN TELLS YOU WHAT YOU NEED TO KNOW
(Johns Hopkins Press Health Book, 1998)
by Lisa Marr
This book presents up-to-date material on 22 STDs

COLOR ATLAS AND SYNOPSIS OF SEXUALLY TRANSMITTED DISEASES
(McGraw-Hill Professional, 2000)
Edited by H. Hunter Handsfield
Really for professionals, this book is a fascinating collection of photos of STD's.

ABC OF SEXUAL HEALTH
(BMJ Books, 1999)
Edited by John Tomlinson
For Doctors, but worth a browse if you get hold of a library copy, as it's up to date with advice on treatment from a UK perspective.

INFORMATION AND ADVICE

Society of Health Advisors in Sexually
Transmitted Diseases
www.shastd.org.uk
Has easy-to-understand information on sexually
transmitted diseases and related conditions, and
where to get help and advice in the UK.

The Terrence Higgins Trust
www.tht.org.uk
The leading HIV and AIDS charity in the UK and
the largest in Europe. It was one of the first
charities to be set up in response to the HIV
epidemic and has been at the forefront of the
fight against HIV and AIDS ever since.

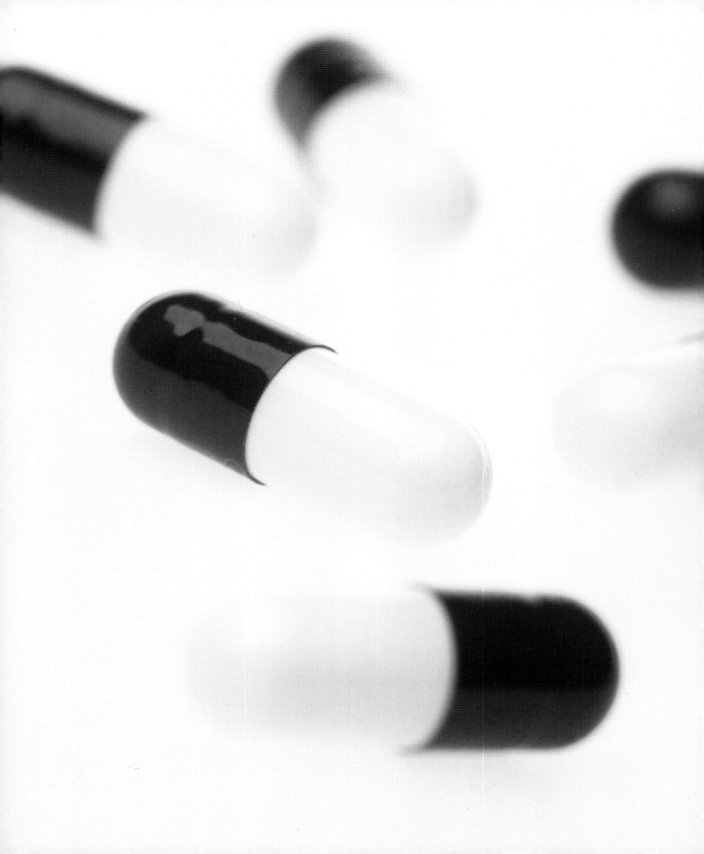

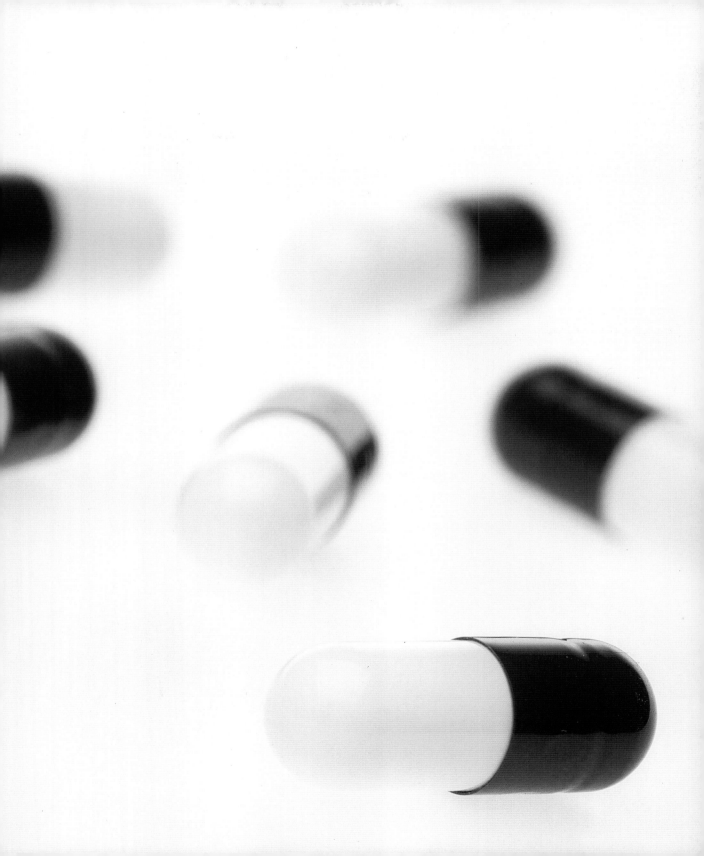

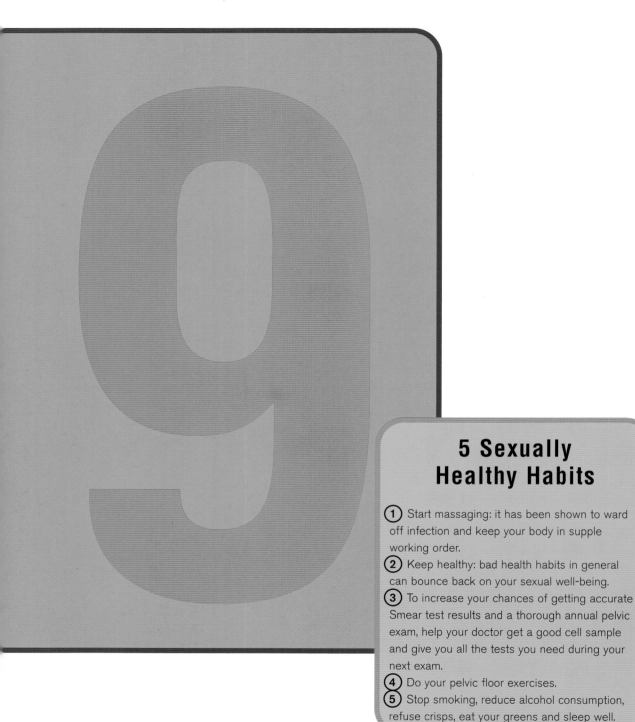

5 Sexually Healthy Habits

(1) Start massaging: it has been shown to ward off infection and keep your body in supple working order.

(2) Keep healthy: bad health habits in general can bounce back on your sexual well-being.

(3) To increase your chances of getting accurate Smear test results and a thorough annual pelvic exam, help your doctor get a good cell sample and give you all the tests you need during your next exam.

(4) Do your pelvic floor exercises.

(5) Stop smoking, reduce alcohol consumption, refuse crisps, eat your greens and sleep well.

EQUIPMENT MAINTENANCE

Everything you need to know about keeping sexually healthy

A big part of keeping yourself sexually healthy – and reaping the benefits of a full sex life – is maintaining your sexual and reproductive health in the first place. You already know that ridding your life of major no-no's like having sex with a new lover without a condom or not getting check-ups can boost your odds of a happier, healthier life sex-wise and generally. But you may be overlooking the little things you do that could jeopardise your sexual health.

Every catastrophe has its warning signs. Your car has a 'check engine' light, your hair dryer starts humming before it breaks down, and your personal CD player beeps at you before its battery runs out. But when it comes to your body, warning signs don't always work. Sometimes they come too late. Sometimes they come disguised as heartburn. And sometimes you simply ignore them, rather than investigating for a closer look. Before long, there's permanent damage.

By paying attention to your sexual health daily, you can get the jump on any problems that may crop up.

It's not really that difficult. Form a few healthy habits, do a little maintenance here and there, run some regular self-checks, and you'll find that your sex system will be built for the long haul.

KEEPING SEXUALLY HEALTHY

Massage has been shown to help ward off infection and keep your body supple, and in general good health. The same goes for sex organ massages. Here are some moves he can give you to keep you in top sexual shape:

- Your cervix is in the upper rear part of your vagina (it feels like a little dome of tissue, and may also have a small cleft in the middle, like your chin). Carefully stimulating the area surrounding the cervix helps keep you lubricated.
- Gently pushing and pulling on the clitoral hood and labia keep them primed for action.
- A hand pressed over the lower part of your abdomen stimulates your sexual chi (energy)
- Gently squeezing a lubricated vaginal lip between the thumb and forefinger while pulling fingers straight away from your body will keep your flexing grip strong.
- Massaging your ovaries (in the deepest part of the vagina to the right or left) helps fertility.

His bad health habits can bounce back on your sexual wellbeing:

- Does he smoke? Besides it affecting his feritlity, there is increasing evidence that spending just one hour inhaling his smoke exposes you to a dose of nitrosamines, increasing your risk of cervical cancer. There is also a connection between the toxins found in a smoking partner's semen and giving birth to a baby with birth defects (if he stops smoking, it takes around 12 weeks for the sperm to be free of chemicals).
- Does he drink? The same types of studies that link a father's smoking to birth defects have shown some similar problems related to paternal drinking.
- Is he a couch potato? Men who burn at least 200 calories a day through exercise are less likely than inactive men to become impotent.

- Does he use a condom? You are more at risk of an STD if he doesn't practise safe sex.
- Does he look after his todger? Does his penis start discharging or burning on its own? 60 per cent of chlamydia cases come with tell-tale symptoms in men as opposed to just 15 per cent in women. So if he ignores tell-tale STD signs, he could infect you and possibly jeopardise your fertility.

Help your doctor to get a good cell sample to increase your chances of getting accurate Smear test results and a thorough pelvic exam.

- Avoid having sex or using tampons within 48 hours of the Smear test (yes, if you do the deed, your doctor can tell – either by the residual semen or by evaluating the vaginal discharge).
- Don't douche (now or ever – see Chapter Two) and don't use vaginal medications or insert spermicide within 72 hours before your examination, because they may remove or obscure abnormal cells.
- Schedule the test for about two weeks after the end of your period.
- Tell your doctor if you've had any abnormal discharge – an infection could trigger a false reading.
- Tell your doctor if you've recently had unprotected and/or high-risk sex, as you may have a symptomless STD which can affect an accurate reading.

Although women are more likely than men to contract an STD from a single exposure, if the man had had the STD diagnosed and treated in the first place, the woman wouldn't have been infected. But men have no equivalent of a yearly pelvic exam. They tend to get investigated when there is a specific problem – such as impotence. This is not good health practice. Studies show that women are diagnosed more often with the silent STDs (see Chapter Seven) because of their annual gynaecological exams.

DO YOU KNOW HOW TO KEEP
HAPPY, HEALTHY & SEXY?

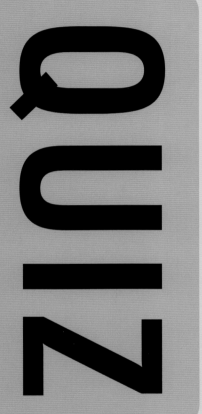

QUESTIONS

postpone menopause and boost your fertility.
e Prevent impotence prostate problems.
f Keep you feeling healthy.
g Make sure you're not alone on Valentine's Day.
h Ensure you get all your zeds.
i Stop you from getting stressed.
j Keep you both alive longer.
k Stop the sniffles.
l Keep the cosmetic surgeon away.
m Increase your breast size.
n Prevent accidental pees.
o Make your boss notice you.

(2) **Folic acid is an important vitamin because it:**
a Prevents an STD.
b Reduces birth defects if you're pregnant.
c Checks vaginal infections.
d Protects your breasts.
e Boosts orgasms.
f Up his sperm count.

(1) **Which of the following won't an orgasm do for you?**
a Give you the body you want.
b Protect you from depression.
c Cure headaches and other pain.
d Regulate your cycle, banish PMS,

(3) **Match the symptom, situation or STD to the test that will be required. Symptoms**
a You had unprotected sex.
b Burning during urination and a frequent need to pee.

c Itching, burning, and/or discharge.
d Red sore or blister.
e Pain during intercourse and painful periods.
f Small bump in genital area.
Required test
i Discharge test.
ii Blood test to detect HIV.
iii Urine test.
iv Smear test.
v Tissue sample.
vi Gynaecological examination.

(4) **Which of the following does not need to be examined monthly?**
a Testicles
b Vulva
c Breasts
d Clitoris
e Penis
f Vagina

(5) **Which of the following edibles is linked to frigidity and a lack of interest in sex (choose one)?**
a Chips fried in vegetable oil.
b Vodka Cosmopolitan
c A take-away burger
d A wedge of Brie

DO YOU KNOW HOW TO KEEP
HAPPY, HEALTHY & SEXY?

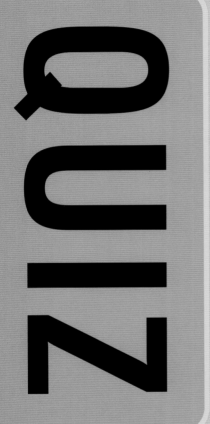

ANSWERS

1 Trick question. An orgasm can do all of the list **(a)** to **(o)**!

(a) Sex is a vigorous form of exercise – your heart and respiratory rates rise and you burn calories.

(b) Sex is an antidepressant, raising the level of serotonin in the brain.

(c) Thanks to the endorphins released during sex, a woman's pain threshold increases substantially during orgasm.

(d) Frequent penile insertions boost levels of the female sex hormone oestrogen, which in turn stimulates your overall reproductive system and keeps it running smoothly.

(e) Frequent erections keep blood flowing through the capillaries, so his wood stays nourished while frequent ejaculations prevent fluid congestion in the prostate gland.

(f) The more sex you have, the more testosterone you're producing which helps the body use energy efficiently, stimulate tissue replacement and bone growth, and promote an overall feeling of wellbeing. The typical orgasm will also boost the body's lymphocyte cells – the cells that fight off foreign invaders.

(g) Oxytocin, a hormone that promotes feelings of intimacy, jumps to five times its normal level during climax.

(h) Oxytocin also induces drowsiness. For women, sleepiness comes about 20 to 30 minutes after orgasm. Men, on the other hand, usually drift off after only two to five minutes.

(i) Stress in women is highly correlated with arousal difficulties, lack of libido and anorgasmia. Just 20 minutes of intercourse, however, releases the lust-enhancing hormone dopamine, triggering a relaxation response that lasts up to two hours.

(j) Men who have two or more orgasms a week tend to live significantly longer than those who have only one or none. Men who have at least three or more orgasms a week are 50 per cent less likely to die from heart failure or coronary heart disease. Women who report being satisfied with their sex lives have a lower incidence of heart ills, cancer, autoimmune disease and infections. From a physiological standpoint, sexual activity increases blood flow to all major organs – not only sexual ones – thus helping keep all systems primed.

(k) Sex twice a week increases levels of Immunoglobulin A (IgA), the most prevalent of the five major human antibodies, which works to neutralise bacteria, flu viruses and other ill-making invaders.

(l) Climaxing temporarily improves your complexion and removes fine wrinkles.

(m) If only for a maximum of a few hours. This is a happy side effect of increased chest-muscle tone and the engorgement caused by heightened blood flow.

(n) Vaginal and pelvic muscles expand and contract during climax, toning them helps them prevent urinary stress-incontinence.

(o) Studies have found a connection between regular sex and fewer sick days off work.

2 Studies have shown that 400 micrograms (0.4 milligrams) daily of the miracle B9 vitamin in folic acid folic may:

(a) Defend against HPV, the STD that increases your risk for genital warts and cervical cancer.

(b) Minimise the risk that your baby will be born with a serious neural tube defect of the spine or brain, when taken prior to conception and during early pregnancy.

(d) Maintain DNA that can be damaged by drinking more than one drink a day (a habit that has been associated with an increased risk of breast cancer).

(e) When combined with zinc supplements, men increased sperm counts by as much as 74 per cent.

3 These are the most likely suspects:

a (ii) You'll need to wait three months for an accurate result. And **(v)** for chlamydia and, if bumps become present, HPV and/or you get red blisters, herpes.

b (iii) to detect UTI or chlamydia.

c (i) to check for vaginitis, or an STD such as BV, gonorrhoea.

d (v) to check for herpes. The sample must be taken from an active sore.

e (vii) to start with, to determine if further investigation is needed for PID and endometriosis.

f (iv) and **(v)** to check for HPV and signs of cervical cancer.

4 Your vagina should be inspected by a gynaecologist yearly to give it a Smear test and an internal examination via the speculum. Vulva and Clitoris Vulval cancer, which affects the external genital area (labia minora or majora or the inner or outer lips of the vulva, respectively) or the clitoris, has been rising for women under 40. The increase may be linked to the growing incidence of HPV. Caught early, vulval cancer is curable in 90 per cent of cases. The key is monthly self-exams:

Use a small mirror to check your outer vaginal area and clitoris. See your doctor if you find any lump patches or red, white or black bumps or if you have persistent itching, pain or inflammation.

Breasts. Early detection and treatment are the best tools currently available in the fight against breast cancer. By age 20, you should be doing exams monthly:

In the shower, when skin is slick and hands can glide smoothly over breast skin, place right hand behind head and use fingertips of left hand to press right breast in a clockwise motion in ever-increasing circles away from the nipples, feeling for lumps and thickening. Repeat on other side.

In front of a mirror, raise both arms overhead then look for swelling, dimpling or discoloration of the skin on breasts or under arms.

Finish by gently squeezing your nipple between your thumb and forefinger to check for clear or milky discharge.

5 (c) Saturated fat content, which s highest in highly processed foods such as fast foods, is linked to frigidity, difficulty reaching orgasm and lack of interest in sex. Cutting back on these foods will help revive and preserve sexual vitality and enhance overall wellbeing.

- Tell your doctor if you take a herbal supplement.
- Let your doctor know if you recently self-treated thrush. It's hard to diagnose yourself and a misdiagnosis can cause your doctor to miss a more serious infection, which can lead to a worsening of symptoms and possibly eventual resistance to treatment (see Chapter Two).
- If it's a new doctor, let them know if you have an STD – some may not be evident when you have your exam (such as HPV, herpes or chlamydia, see Chapter Eight).
- Make your doctor aware if you find sex painful. Your lack of pleasure may be due to a treatable physical problem, such as a medication you are taking, endometriosis, fibroids, cysts or PID.
- 'Fess up if you haven't followed doctor's orders. The doctor needs to know if you haven't taken the full course of your prescribed antibiotics for thrush, because it means you may have only killed the weak bugs and ended up breeding a colony of strong ones that stick with you.

Do your pelvic floor exercises: Studies have found that flexing the pubococcygeus (PC) muscle during intercourse brings more blood flow to the vagina, heightening sensitivity and upgrading the chance and pleasure factor of an orgasm. In fact, you can jumpstart a powerful orgasm by pushing the PC muscle outward just as you verge on climax – the jolt of the voluntary spasm intensifies the involuntary contractions that follow.

Pelvic floor exercises also keep the vaginal area primed and help avoid urinary incontinence and vaginal prolapse (common after pregnancy) in women and erection droops in men. It may take up to 100 pelvic floor exercises daily for a few weeks before you notice any improvement in tone, but it's well worth getting into the habit.

Here's how to do them correctly:

- Find your PC muscles. In men, they anchor the base of his penis several inches within the pelvis, in women, they surround the vaginal wall. These three sets of muscles run from the back to front of your pubic bone, encircling the openings of the vagina and rectum. The easiest way to locate them is to try to stop your urine flow while on the loo (don't do this more than once a day, as it may aggravate your bladder). You could insert a finger in your vagina or place your hand at the opening to detect the movement and confirm that you are squeezing the correct muscles.

Once you have a general idea of that feeling, practise the basic pelvic floor exercise:

- With legs slightly apart (rather than with thighs clamped together), squeeze your pelvic floor muscle and hold for a count of five. If at first, you may not be able to hold it more than a second or two, don't worry. With practice, you should be able to tighten the muscles for ten seconds or more. Remember to relax for ten seconds or so before contracting your pelvic floor muscles again.
- Vary this with quickly contracting the pelvic muscles several times in succession. Both of these exercise types can be done practically any time, anywhere.

A few lifestyle tweaks can quickly help you to better sexual health – and the best sex ever.

- Stop smoking: lighting up can stop you from

> Pelvic floor exercises are surprisingly easy to flub. Only half the women in one study did the exercises correctly. One quarter did them in a way that not only was useless but might have increased their risk of incontinence. The most common, and damaging, pelvic floor mistake is to contract the abs instead of, or along with, the pelvic muscles. This increases the pressure on your abdomen and actually opens the urethra, promoting leakage. To keep your abs relaxed, press gently on your belly so you'll feel if you contract those muscles. A hint: If you're holding your breath or you find Pelvic floor exercises tiring, you're probably squeezing your abs.

climaxing, him from getting an erection, you from going on the Pill and getting pregnant.

- Aim for a healthy weight: shedding excess pounds can make you feel sexier and increase blood circulation, making orgasm more likely.
- Watch your alcohol intake: an occasional glass or two is fine, but climax quality diminishes when you've had too much to drink, and more than one drink daily has been connected with increased breast cancer risk (see Chapter One).

> If you think you have a vaginal infection, you need a swab to get samples of discharge. It's important to mention any unusual discharge or odour to your doctor because some unchecked infections can lead to PID. The Smear test checks for changes in the cells of your cervix to detect cervical cancer or precancerous conditions – abnormalities of the cervix that may lead to cancer (see Chapter Two).

- Decline the crisps: downing high-fat foods leads to clogged arteries, which makes it harder for blood to circulate to all parts of your body, including your V zone.
- Put yourself to bed: and get enough shut-eye. Sex hormone levels – and consequently your libido – may take a nosedive if you're walking around sleep-deprived.
- Hop off the couch: regular exercise can boost your libido by increasing the levels of endorphins and sex hormones in your body.
- Eat greens: asparagus and avocados contain niacin, which may trigger sexual sensation, while broccoli has vitamin B5, which aids sex hormone production.
- Try to get over any hang-ups about masturbation: regular orgasms are good for you, however you make them happen (see quiz on p.210j21).
- Take your tests: BSE and vulvar once a month, gynaecological and Smear test once a year and STDs if you have unsafe sex.
- Ask questions about your family history: sexual

- health disorders may also be genetic.
- Use a condom (see Chapters Eight and Six) unless you are in a monogamous safe relationship.

BOOKS

THE GREAT SEX WEEKEND: A 48-HOUR GUIDE TO REKINDLING SPARKS FOR BOLD, BUSY, OR BORED LOVERS: INCLUDES A 24-HOUR PLAN FOR THE REALLY BUSY
(Putman Pub Group, 1998)
by Pepper Schwartz and Janet Lever
Experts Pepper Schwartz and Janet Lever offer no magical elixirs of youth, just a weekend guide to re-ignited love, road-tested by diligent researchers, with specifics on how to partake of a weekend away that's devoted to recovering intimacy and the pleasures of the flesh.

GREAT SEX FOR LIFE: ESSENTIAL TECHNIQUES
(Hamlyn, 1997)
by Linda Sonntag
This straight-talking guide for modern lovers is packed with practical advice that will help keep your love life simmering 365 days a year.

THE BUSY COUPLE'S GUIDE TO GREAT SEX: THE MEDICALLY PROVEN PROGRAM TO BOOST LOW LIBIDO
(Running Press Book Publishers, 2004)
by Rallie McAllister
Author Rallie McAllister, a board-certified family physician, gives a medically credible approach to low libido, examining contributing factors such as hormone imbalance, tobacco and alcohol use, specific prescription drugs, conflicts within the relationship, and body image with explanations on how to resolve each one. The book also features an 'aphrodisiac diet', with recipes and menus to boost energy levels and maximise performance, plus a 'sexual fitness' programme.

THE BETTER SEX DIET: THE MEDICALLY BASED LOW-FAT EATING PLAN FOR INCREASED SEXUAL VITALITY IN JUST 6 WEEKS
(St. Martin's Press, 1996)
by Lynn Fischer
Good health is an essential part of good sex. This expert guide translates the latest scientific facts into delicious recipes that will enhance sexual vitality naturally in just six weeks.

INFORMATION AND ADVICE

www.askthecouch.com
For a sex advice column that covers much of the
nitty and gritty of your sex and relationship
questions go to this website.

The Sexual Health infoCenter
www.sexhealth.org
Provides information and forums for adults to
discuss human sexuality and it's nuances.

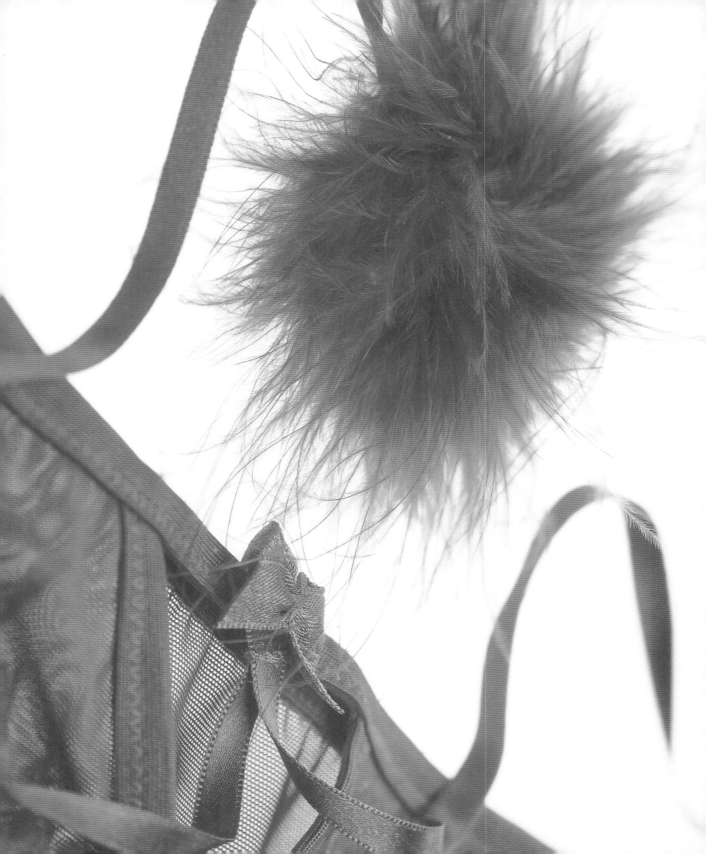

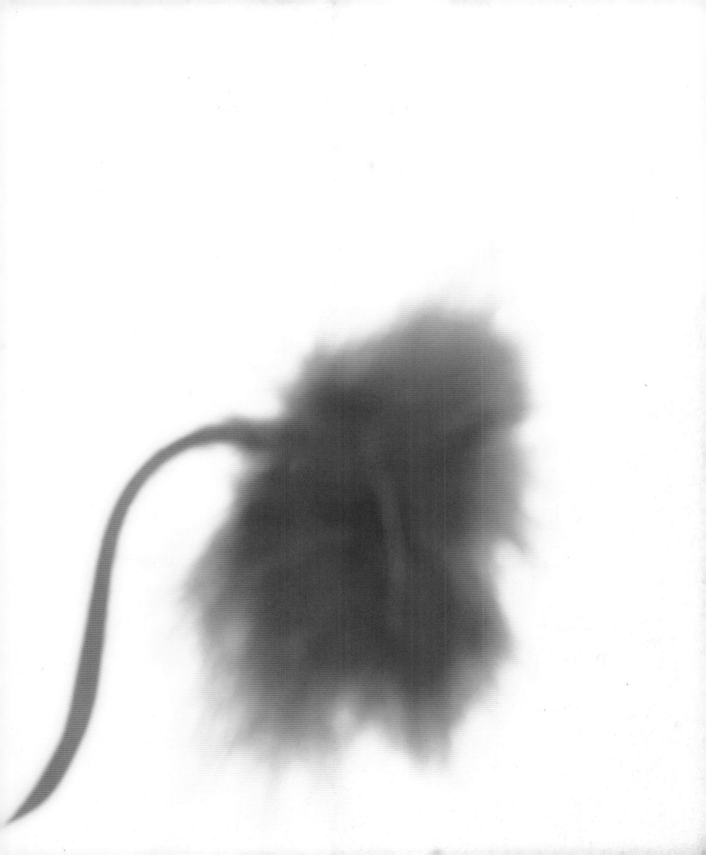

INDEX

A huge thank you to the many medical professionals, organisations, journals and institutions who generously shared their time, expertise and vast knowledge and ensured that my information was accurate and up-to-date. Thanks to:

Alan Guttmacher Institute

American College of Obstetrics and
    Gynecology

The Brooks Institute

British Journal of Obstetrics and Gynaecology

Centers for Disease Control and Prevention

Department of Health (UK)

The Family Planning Association

Harvard Medical School

Henry J Kaiser Family Foundation

International Society on the Preventative
    Aspects of Infertility

The Kinsey Institute

Masters and Johnson

National Cancer Institute

National Endometriosis Society

Planned Parenthood Federation of America

Royal College of Obstetricians and
    Gynaecologists

The World Health Organization

And last, but certainly not least, this book could not have been written without the insight, patience, know-how and tactful touch of Victoria Alers-Hankey, the support of Emma Dally, Heather Welford's generous input and advice, the incredible (and incredibly inexpensive) research abilities of Sy Sussman, the statistical know-how and patience of Steven Moss and the silly jokes from Jazz and Tasha. Without you, there would be no book at all.

PICTURE CREDITS

page 6, 216-17 Thanks to the online store: **www.gash.co.uk** – award winning designer of lingerie and erotica

pages 2, 10–11, 30-31, 92–93 Thanks to Myla: **www.myla.com**